SO-EJQ-638

UC San Francisco LIBRARY

UNIVERSITY OF CALIFORNIA

ANTHRACYCLINES

Current Status and
Future Developments

Edited by
Georges Mathé, M.D.
René Maral, M.D.
Robert De Jager, M.D.

UNIVERSITY OF CALIFORNIA
SAN FRANCISCO
LIBRARY

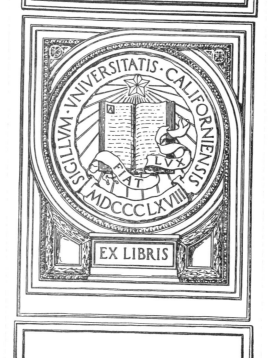

EX LIBRIS

ANTHRACYCLINES

Current Status and Future Developments

edited by

Georges Mathé, M.D.

Service de Malades Sanguines et
Tumorales, Hôpital Universitaire Paul-Brousse;
Institut de Cancérologie et d'Immunogénétique
(ICIG), Villejuif, France

René Maral, M.D.

Institut de Cancérologie et d' Immunogénétique
(ICIG), Villejuif, France

Robert De Jager, M.D.

Unite de Pharmacologie Clinique des Cancers
Foundation Simone et Cino del Duca (ICIG)
Paris, France

RC271
A63
A568
1983

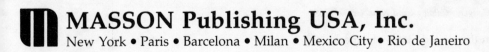

MASSON Publishing USA, Inc.
New York • Paris • Barcelona • Milan • Mexico City • Rio de Janeiro

Proceedings of the International Symposium on Tumor Pharmacotherapy, sponsored by the Simone and Cino Del Duca Foundation, Paris, France, 1981.

Library of Congress Cataloging in Publication Data

Main entry under title:

Anthracyclines, 1981.

   Papers of a symposium of the Fondation Simone et Cino Del Duca held in Paris, June 24-25, 1981.
Bibliography: p.
Includes index.
1. Cancer—Chemotherapy—Congresses.
2. Anthracyclines—Testing—Congresses. I. Mathé,
Georges, 1922-   . II. De Jager, Robert. III. Maral,
Rene. IV. Fondation Simone et Cino Del Duca.
[DNLM: 1. Antibiotics, Antineoplastic—Congresses.
QV 269 A628 1981]
RC271.A63A568 1982   616.99′4061   82-12691
ISBN 0-89352-188-4   Rev.

Copyright © 1983 by Masson Publishing USA, Inc.

All rights reserved. No part of this book may be reproduced in any form, by photostat, microform, retrieval system, or any other means, without the prior written permission of the publisher.

ISBN 0-89352-188-4
Library of Congress Catalog Card Number: 82-12691

Printed in the United States of America

PREFACE

When Madame Cino Del Duca spoke to me of her wish to do something for research, as applied to the health of Man, I suggested "Human Cancer Pharmacology," a subject about which she was highly enthusiastic.

The members of her Foundation's Scientific Council, while not giving a clear-cut opinion, understood her enthusiasm for this subject and advised her to visit the Institut de Cancérologie et d'Immunogénétique in Villejuif and to make the final decision herself.

She listened attentively to my arguments for the urgent need to develop the ICIG, an Institute where research ranges from basic molecular biology to human medical oncology and after having seen the patients, both adults and children, receiving chemotherapy without the scientific groundwork which could increase activity and reduce risk, she rapidly reached a decision to create the Unité de Pharmacologie Cellulaire et Moléculaire et de Pharmacocinétique, the achievement which will only be evaluable after three years.

We intended to set up pharmacology at the molecular, cell, tissue, organ, and total body levels for cytostatics during the first year and for biological response modifiers during the second year. From September 1980 to September 1981, we started the first program and studied agents belonging to three series. First, aclacinomycin A, an analogue of the anthracycline family, isolated by H. Umezawa (to whom this meeting is devoted), and compared to other derivatives of this series; Second, several nitrosourea derivatives of French origin (Imbach and Montero) were compared to other French analogues of this drug family (RFCNU, RPCNU), to a German analogue, to HECFU, and to the American chlorozotocin; finally, another French compound (Potier and Langlois), navelbine, which is a new semi-synthetic Vinca alkaloid, was compared to the two older Vinca alkaloids, vinblastine and vincristine, and to the more recent one, vindesine.

The program for 1981–1982 will be devoted to the development in Man of the "biological response modifiers" (BRM), which we have already studied in animals and Man, but without a developed scientific pharmacological approach.

We are interested in: two immunomodifiers—azimexon and tuftsin; bestatin, a compound discovered by Umezawa, which we have shown to be able to restore the immune functions in aged mice and that simultaneously prevents spontaneous tumors caused by aging; and agents acting both on the tumor cells (on division and differentiation) and on the immune and other cell populations involved in homeostatic phenomena. These include several interferons (and other lymphoid cytokines, lymphokines) and several retinoids which have been shown experimentally to exert an anticarcinogenic effect, an effect which we have confirmed in humans, showing, after systematic bronchial fibroscopy, that precancerous metaplasia is very strong among smokers and that a 6-month treatment with a retinoid can induce its disappearance.

In this field, of course, the administration of these agents (BRM) to humans seems less dangerous than with the cytostatics. However, we need more scientific information in pharmacology to render the use of these compounds more active and better tolerated in human therapeutics.

Georges Mathé, M.D.

FOREWORD

Homage to Professor H. Umezawa

Everybody knows Hamao Umezawa as the therapeutic chemist who has created an enormous number of useful agents for health and life, such as 70 antimicrobial antibiotics, the best known being kanamycin (1957); 30 antitumor antibiotics — the most well-known are bleomycin (1953), aclacinomycin (1974), pepleomycin (1976), and THP-adriamycin (1979); immunity adjuvants, the most interesting is bestatin; and compounds useful in other fields of human problems, for example, kasugamycin (1976), which is used in the prevention of a rice plant disease.

This tremendous productivity, while indicating the incomparable efficiency of Umezawa and the Japanese, might lead those who have not followed his work to think that he is only a fortunate and hard-working researcher, greatly helped by a large group of good co-workers. However, as with the greatest artists' achievements, there is, in Umezawa's contribution, a biological and even a philosophical approach to a complete technical mastership.

Let us follow his progress: Hamao Umezawa was impressed by the discovery of Florey, Chain, and Abraham of the antibacterial effect of penicillin in 1941, and by that of Waksman of streptomycin, in 1943. He entered the field of microbial secondary metabolites in 1944 with two objectives. The first was to search for a great number of "bacterial antibiotics," because the few available were far from capable of curing all infectious diseases and he predicted that germs sensitive to them would become resistant. His second objective was a search for antitumor antibiotics. As far as the first objective is concerned, he personally contributed greatly to the solution. In 1957 he discovered Kanamycin, which works in many infections that are resistant to classical antibiotics. Moreover, he carefully studied the appearance of resistance to Kanamycin and clarified the enzymatic mechanism of the aminoglycosidic-resistant antibiotics, predicting chemical structures of derivatives which would be active against resistant organisms; this approach opened the way to the synthesis of such agents, by himself, of Dibecacin, and by others of, Amikacin.

In the field of antitumor antibiotics, he discovered many agents in microbial culture filtrates. Bleomycin is the first antitumor agent which is neither myelotoxic, immunosuppressive, nor mutagenic, and which is able to cure certain tumors such as skin tumors inaccessible to surgery or radiotherapy. Bleomycin is also of help in curing other malignancies, such as tumors of the testes. It is Umezawa who suggested to the clinicians the tumors to be submitted to Bleomycin, because they arose from tissues poor in Bleomycin Hydrolase.

The antagonistic effect of this antibiotic on DNA repair, in conjunction with its lack of myelo- and immunotoxicity, makes it one of the most important cytostatics for modern combinations used in medical treatment of cancer. Umezawa recently prepared an analogue, pepleomycin, which is better tolerated; however, cross-resistance between them has to be studied.

Among one of the last antitumor antibiotics discovered by Umezawa is aclacinomycin, which has already given us very impressive results in acute myeloid and lymphoid leukemia, and in leukemic non-Hodgkin's lymphoma. In a phase II trial, we are currently clinically studying pepleomycin, which has given very encouraging results, and are conducting a phase I trial on THP-adriamycin which is—with aclacinomycin—in our study in hamsters, one of the least toxic compounds among the anthracyclines for hair and the myocardium.

Soon after we started cancer immunotherapy, Umezawa was well aware of the impossible situation of therapists who had to conduct a modern war with a Middle Age weapon such as BCG. He decided to help us and to contribute to the Renaissance period of immunotherapy by preparing immunity adjuvants which could be used in a satisfactory and identical quantitative manner in Great Britain or France, for example. He had noticed that aminopeptidases were present on the surface of various cells and not released extracellularly. He assumed that such substances might play a role in immune processes and studied the effect on immune functions of bestatin, an inhibitor of aminopeptidases B and leucine-aminopeptidases. Bestatin was shown, in Japan, to exert some effect on delayed HST. Since we had shown that 18- to 24-month-old mice of nonleukemogenic or tumorigenic strains presented several immune markers and 30% late neoplasias, mainly non-Hodgkin's lymphomas, we studied, with M. Bruley-Rosset and I. Florentin, the effect of bestatin on these aged mice. We induced immunorestoration and prevented the appearance of late tumors related to aging.

Observing that the production of an antibiotic is restricted to certain microbial strains, but not to certain species, and that a given antibiotic may be produced by several microbial species, Umezawa thought that plasmids were involved in the biosynthesis of antibiotics. For example, he found that the production of Kasugamycin (an agent he discovered and used in the prevention of a rice plant disease) was arrested when using certain culture media in which plasmids were eliminated. He confirmed his original discovery on the role of plasmids with the study of other antibiotics.

He also confirmed the involvement of plasmids in the biosynthesis of antibiotics by genetic analysis of recombinants formed by crossing Chloramphenicol-producing and nonproducing mutants. This same year he isolated plasmids related to the production of Kasugamycin or to Aureothricin. One year later, he showed that a plasmid was involved in the biosynthesis of a structural moiety of the molecule. He succeeded in transferring the ability to biosynthetize Leucopeptin acid from a Leucopeptin mutant to a nonproducing mutant.

This method of conducting research distinguishes a man of genius from a man of mere talent. This is why I recognize something in Umezawa's work that I do not recognize in the work of many therapeutic chemists, in the same way that I recognize in a work of art by Raphael or Michelangelo that which I do not find among thousands of paintings or statues in a museum.

But people of genius do still more—they help human beings to understand life. From Umezawa's work on plasmids, one conceives that molecular changes due to mutations may cause production of new secondary metabolites which, in the natural environment, may change the microbiological flora. These changes may not only automatically directly affect the population of the other microorganisms, but they may induce mutations since many secondary metabolites are mutagenic, and thus change the production of such metabolites eventually affecting the flora.

The impact of these thoughts in microorganic ecology and its possible influence on all living organic ecosociology suggests the role of interconnections between living organisms.

Hence, Umezawa's basic discoveries have not only produced applications which are extremely useful both directly and indirectly to the well-being of humans, but they are already contributing the answer to some fundamental philosophical questions about the evolution of life.

Georges Mathé, M.D.

CONTRIBUTORS

E. Acton, Life Sciences Division, SRI International, Menlo Park, California

I. Amaki, First Department of Internal Medicine, Nagoya University, School of Medicine, Showa-ku, Nagoya, Japan

C. Andrade-Mena, Institut de Cancerologie et d'Immunogénétique, Hôpital Universitaire Paul-Brousse, Villejuif, France

F. Arcamone, Ricerca and Sviluppo Chimico-Farmitalia Carlo Erba, Milano, Italy

M.F. Auclerc, Service d'Oncologie Médicale, Hôpital de la Salpetrière, Paris, France

N.R. Bachur, Laboratory of Clinical Biochemistry, Baltimore Cancer Research Program, Division of Cancer Treatment, National Cancer Institute, NIH

R. Baurain, International Institute of Cellular and Molecular Pathology, and Université Cathologique of Luvain, Brussels, Belgium

M. Bennoun, Institut de Cancérologie et d'Immunogénétique, Hôpital Universitaire Paul-Brousse, Villejuif, France

J. Bernard, Service d'Oncologie Médicale, Hôpital de la Salpetrière, Paris, France

V. Bonfante, Istituto Nazionale Tumori, Milan, Italy

C. Bonnet, Service de Pharmacologie, Faculté de Médecine Pitié Salpetrière, Paris, France

C.E. Bourut, Institut de Cancérologie et d'Immunogénétique, Hôpital Universitaire Paul-Brousse, U-50 INSERM, Villejuif, France

R.J. Brooks, University of Arizona, Cancer Center, Tucson, Arizona

C.G. Caillard, Centre de Recherches Nicolas Grillet, Rhône Poulenc, Vitry sur Seine, France

A.M. Casazza, Farmitalia Carlo Erba Research Laboratories, Milan, Italy

D. Dantchev, Institut de Cancérologie et d'Immunogénétique, Hôpital Universitaire Paul-Brousse, Villejuif, France

R. De Jager, Institut de Cancérologie et d'Immunogénétique, Hôpital Universitaire Paul Brousse, Villejuif, France

M. Delgado, Institut de Cancérologie et d'Immunogénétique, Hôpital Unviersitaire Paul Brousse, Villejuif, France

M. Denechaud, Laboratoire de Physique Nucléaire Appliquée et Radiobiologie, Université de Bordeaux II, Bordeaux, France

D. Deprez-De Campeneere, International Institute of Cellular and Molecular Pathology, and Université Catholique of Luvain, Brussels, Belgium

M.M. De Planque, Clinical Research Unit, Department of Internal Medicine, Antoni van Leeuwenhoekhuis, Netherlands Cancer Institute, Amsterdam, the Netherlands

F. De Vassal, Institut de Cancérologie et d'Immunogénétique, Hôpital Universitaire Paul-Brousse, Villejuif, France

A. Di Marco, Division of Experimental Oncology B Istituto Nazionale per lo Studio et la Cura dei Tumori, Milan, Italy

B. Diquet, Service de Pharmacologie, Faculté de Médecine Pitié Salpetrière, Paris, France

J.P. Emond, Department of Biochemistry, Faculty of Medicine, Laval University, Quebec, Canada

A. Fourcade, Institut de Cancérologie et d'Immunogénétique, Hôpital Universitaire Paul-Brousse, Villejuif, France

G. Gahrton, Section of Clinical Hematology, Department of Medicine, Huddinge Hospital, Huddinge, Sweden

P. Ganter, Centre de Recherches Nicolas Grillet, Rhône Poulenc, Vitry Sur Seine, France

J. Gastiaburu, Institut de Cancérologie et d'Immunogénétique, Hôpital Universitaire Paul-Brousse, Villejuif, France.

M.A. Gil-Delgado, Institut de Cancérologie et d'Immunogénétique, Hôpital Universitaire Paul Brousse, Villejuif, France

G.M. Ginsbourg, Institut de Cancérologie et d'Immunogénétique, Hôpital Universitaire Paul-Brousse, Villejuif, France

F. Giuliani, Division of Experimental Oncology B Istituto Nazionale per lo Studio et la Cura dei Tumori, Milan, Italy

A. Goldin, Division of Cancer Treatment, N.C.I., Bethesda, Maryland

J. Gouveia, Institut de Cancérologie et d'Immunogénétique, Hôpital Universitaire Paul-Brousse, Villejuif, France

Group Inter France, Institut de Cancérologie et d'Immunogénétique, Villejuif, France

M. Hayat, Institut de Cancérologie et d'Immunogénétique, Hôpital Universitaire Paul Brousse, Villejuif, France

T.S. Herman, Department of Internal Medicine, Section of Hematology/Oncology, University of Arizona College of Medicine, Tucson, Arizona

Y. Hirota, First Department of Internal Medicine, Nagoya University, School of Medicine, Showa-ku, Nagoya, Japan

B. Hoerni, Fondation Bergonié, Bordeaux, France.

R. Hulhoven, Laboratory of Pharmacotherapy, Catholic University of Louvain, Brussels, Belgium

P. Hurteloup, Centre Hospitalier et Universitaire, Service de Radiothérapie, Besançon, France

J. Inagaki, First Department of Internal Medicine, Nagoya University, School of Medicine, Showa-ku, Nagoya, Japan

M. Ito, First Department of Internal Medicine, Nagoya University, School of Medicine, Showa-ku, Nagoya, Japan

Cl. Jacquillat, Service d'Oncologie Médicale, Hôpital de la Salpetrière, Paris, France

Cl. Jasmin, Institut de Cancérologie et d'Immunogénétique, Hôpital Universitaire Paul-Brousse, Villejuif, France

R.A. Jensen, Life Sciences Division, SRI International, Menlo Park, California

L. Julou, Centre de Recherches Nicolas Grillet, Rhône Poulenc, Vitry Sur Seine, France

N.O. Kaplan Department of Chemistry and the Cancer Center, University of California at San Diego, La Jolla, California

J. Khayat, Service de Pharmacologie, Faculté de Médecine Pitié Salpetrière, Paris, France

T. Kitahara, First Department of Internal Medicine, Nagoya University, School of Medicine, Showa-ku, Nagoya, Japan

S. Kurita, First Department of Internal Medicine, Nagoya University, School of Medicine, Showa-ku, Nagoya, Japan

T.J. Lampidis, Signey Farber Cancer Institute, Boston, Massachusetts

M. Laval, Laboratoire de Physique Nucléaire Appliquée et Radiobiologie, Université de Bordeaux II, Bordeaux, France

D. Machover, Institut de Canceérologie et d'Immunogénétique, Hôpital Universitaire Paul-Brousse, Villejuif, France

T. Maekawa, First Department of Internal Medicine, Nagoya University, School of Medicine, Showa-ku, Nagoya, Japan

J. Maral, Service d'Oncologie Médicale, Hôpital de la Salpetrière, Paris, France

R. Maral, Institut de Cancérologie et d'Immunogénétique, Hôpital Universitaire Paul-Brousse, Villejuif, France

J.P. Marie, Service d'Hématologie de l'Hôtel-Dieu, Paris, France

T. Masaoka, First Department of Internal Medicine, Nagoya University, School of Medicine, Showa-ku, Nagoya, Japan

M. Masquelier, International Institute of Cellular and Molecular Pathology, and Université Catholique of Louvain, Brussels, Belgium

G. Mathe, Institut de Cancérologie et d'Immunogénétique, Hôpital Universitaire Paul-Brousse, Villejuif, France

E. Mc Culloch, Ontario Cancer Institute, Toronto, Canada

J.G. McVie, Clinical Research Unit, Department of Internal Medicine, Antoni van Leeuwenhoekhuis Netherlands Cancer Institute, Amsterdam, the Netherlands

P. Michaux, Hôpital Saint Luc, U.C.L., Brussels, Belgium

J.L. Misset, Institut de Cancérologie et d'Immunogénétique, Hôpital Universitaire Paul-Brousse, Villejuif, France

S. Mondot, Centre de Recherches Nicolas Grillet, Rhône Poulenc, Vitry sur Seine, France

T. Nakamura, First Department of Internal Medicine, Nagoya University, School of Medicine, Showa-ku, Nagoya, Japan

N. Nakano, First Department of Internal Medicine, Nagoya University, School of Medicine, Showa-ku, Nagoya, Japan

R.A. Newman, Vermont Regional Cancer Center, Department of Pharmacology, College of Medicine, University of Vermont, Burlington, Vermont

M. Oguro, First Department of Internal Medicine, Nagoya University, School of Medicine, Showa-ku, Nagoya, Japan

T. Oki, Central Research Laboratories, Sanraku Ocean Company, Fujisawa, Japan

K. Onozawa, First Department of Internal Medicine, Nagoya University, School of Medicine, Showa-ku, Nagoya, Japan

S. Orbach-Arbouys, Institut de Cancérologie et d'Immunogénétique, Hôpital Universitaire Paul-Brousse, Villejuif, France

S. Osamura, First Department of Internal Medicine, Nagoya University, School of Medicine, Showa-ku, Nagoya, Japan

M. Page, Department of Biochemistry, Faculty of Medicine, Laval University, Quebec, Canada

M. Paintrand, Institut de Cancérologie et d'Immunogénétique, Hôpital Universitaire Paul-Brousee, Villejuif, France

J. Pasquet, Centre de Recherches Nicolas Grillet, Rhône Poulenc, Vitry Sur Seine, France

C. Paul, Section of Clinical Hematology, Department of Medicine, Huddinge Hospital, Huddinge, Sweden

J.H. Peters, Life Sciences Division, SRI International, Menlo Park, California

C. Peterson, Department of Pharmacology, Karolinska Institute, Stockholm, Sweden

I. Pignot, Institut de Cancérologie et d'Immunogénétique, Hôpital Universitaire Paul Brousse, Villejuif, France

A. Rahman, Division of Medical Oncology School of Medicine, Vincent T. Lobardi Cancer Research Center, Georgetown University Hospital, Washington, DC

P. Ribaud, Institut de Cancérologie et d'Immunogénétique, Hôpital Universitaire Paul Brousse, Villejuif, France

J. Robert, Fondation Bergonié, Bordeaux, France

P.S. Schein, Department of Chemistry and the Cancer Center, University of California at San Diego, La Jolla, California

L. Schwarzenberg, Institut de Cancérologie et d'Immunogénétique, Hôpital Universitaire Paul Brousse, Villejuif, France

P. Simon, Service de Pharmacologie, Faculté de Médecine Pitié Salpetrière, Paris, France

G.P.C. Simonetti, Clinical Research Unit, Department of Internal Medicine, Antoni van Leeuwenhoekhuis Netherlands Cancer Institute, Amsterdam, the Netherlands

G. Sokal, Hôpital Saint Luc, U.C.L., Brussels, Belgium

H. Takaku, First Department of Internal Medicine, Nagoya University, School of Medicine, Showa-ku, Nagoya, Japan

H. Tapiero, Institut de Cancérologie et d'Immunogénétique, Hôpital Universitaire Paul-Brousee, Villejuif, France

W.W. ten Bokkel Huinink, Clinical Research Unit, Department of Internal Medicine, Antoni van Leeuwenhoekhuis Netherlands Cancer Institute, Amsterdam, the Netherlands

A. Trouet, International Institute of Cellular and Molecular Pathology, and Université Catholique of Louvain, Brussels, Belgium

T. Tsuruo, First Department of Internal Medicine, Nagoya University, School of Medicine, Showa-ku, Nagoya, Japan

H. Umezawa, Microbial Chemistry Research Institute, Tokyo, Japan

Y. Uzuka, First Department of Internal Medicine, Nagoya University, School of Medicine, Showa-ku, Nagoya, Japan

M. Weil, Service d'Oncologie Médicale, Hôpital de la Salpetrière, Paris, France

K. Yamada, First Department of Internal Medicine, Nagoya University, School of Medicine, Showa-ku, Nagoya, Japan

G. Zbinden, Institute of Toxicology Swiss Federal Institute of Technology, and University of Zurich, Schwerzenbach, Switzerland

R. Zittoun, Service d'Hématologie de l'Hôtel-Dieu, Paris, France

CONTENTS

Part V. Clinical Studies: Classical Agents

Part VI. Clinical Studies: New Agents

Part I

Experimental Activity and Toxicity

CHAPTER 1

Experimental Activity

R. Maral*

Many hundreds of analogues of dauno-rubicin (DNR)[1] and of doxorubicin (DOX) or adriamycin (ADM)[2] have been synthesized during the last 20 years. The aim of research in this field is to find new derivatives that have

1. Broader spectrum and higher antitumor activity
2. Lower toxicity, principally a less cardiotoxic effect
3. Different pharmacokinetics
4. No cross-resistance with the parent compounds

The main anthracycline analogues of which clinical activity has been or is presently under evaluation are zorubicin, or rubidazone,[3] and detorubicin[4] from France; 4'-epi-DOX from Italy[5]; AD-32[6] and, more recently, AD-143 from the United States; aclacinomycin A[7] and the tetrahydropyranyl derivative of DOX (THP-ADM)[8] from Japan; and carminomycin from the Soviet Union[9] (see Fig. 1). Many other semisynthetic derivatives have been synthesized, principally by reactions on the aglycone moiety and on the amino and the keto groups of DNR or DOX.[10,11]

The aim of the experimental activity studies is not only to find active derivatives, but, above all, to find compounds that are clearly superior in activity and, at the same time, are low in toxicity compared to the parent compounds. It should be emphasized that the arguments for starting clinical evaluation of an analogue are more complex than the decision to test a new compound with a new structure.

The methods (in vitro and in vivo) currently used for screening and studying the activities of compounds should be reexamined; these methods need to be improved because it is not known how predictive the routine systems are for categorically stating an analogue's superiority.

In this chapter we will review the different systems at our disposal for the selection of an analogue, and we will examine the need for improved methods of studying the efficacy of analogues experimentally with a view to better clinical predictions.

In vitro Studies

With this class of compound, in vitro studies may be of some help, principally for determining the doses to be used in vivo.[12]

CYTOTOXICITY IN TISSUE CULTURE

Different cell strains are used:

1. Normal cells (for example, primary fibroblast cultures), comparison of sensitivity with immortalized analogue cells
2. Malignant cell strains, such as KB, HeLa, or L1210
3. Chemical or viral transformed cells

The cytolysis follows first-order kinetics, and the inhibiting concentration (IC_{50}) is graphically established. The cell population is studied by various means, for example, Coulter cell numeration, cell protein dos-

Institut de Cancérologie et d'Immunogénétique (I.C.I.G.) et Hôpital Universitaire Paul-Brousse, Villejuif Cédex, France

3

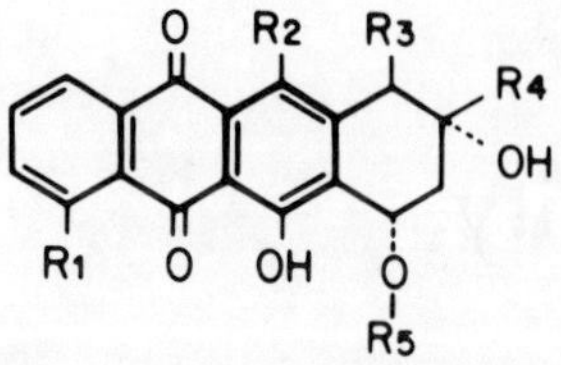

COMPOUND	R1	R2	R3	R 4	R 5
Adriamycin (Doxorubicin)(ADM)	-OCH₃	-OH	-H₂	-CO CH₂ OH	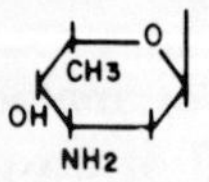 (sugar: CH₃, OH, NH₂)
Daunorubicin (DNR)	-OCH₃	-OH	-H₂	-CO CH₃	-id-
Rubidazone (Zorubicin)(RBZ)	-OCH₃	-OH	-H₂	-C(CH₃)NNHCOC₆H₅	-id-
Detorubicin (DTR)	-OCH₃	-OH	-H₂	-CO CH₂OCOCH(OC₂H₅)₂	-id-
4'epi-Adriamycin (e-ADM)	-OCH₃	-OH	-H₂	-COCH₂OH	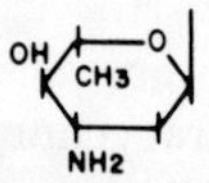 (sugar: OH, CH₃, NH₂)
AD-32	-OCH₃	-OH	-H₂	-COCH₂OCO(CH₂)₃CH₃	(sugar: CH₃, OH, NHCOCF₃)
Aclacinomycin A (ACM)	-OH	-H	-COOCH₃	-CH₂CH₃	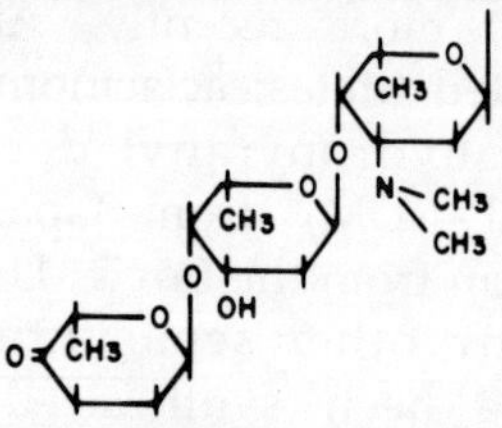 (trisaccharide: CH₃, CH₃, N(CH₃)₂, OH, O=C-CH₃)

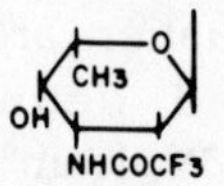

FIGURE 1. The main anthracycline analogues whose clinical activity has been or is being evaluated.

age, and cytofluorograph numeration of dead cells. Another comparative technique is the diffusion in agar of the drugs over a layer of cell culture.[13]

SPECIAL TECHNIQUES

Due to the technical complexity, *organotypic cultures* have not often been used for the comparative studies of anthracyclines.

Differential sensitivity of human tumor stem cells, according to the Salmon technique,[14] may be an important help in comparing the activities. However, much work has to be devoted to this topic in the future.

The detection in culture of the ability of analogues to *induce differentiation* in various myeloid leukemic cell clones, according to the technique of Leo Sachs,[15] may be a new means of selecting analogues. We know that DOX is an inducer of differentiation, but it is weaker than actinomycin D.

In vivo **Studies**

GRAFTED TUMORS

Sarcomas (fibrosarcomas, rhabdomyosarcomas, osteosarcomas), carcinomas (Lewis lung carcinoma, B16 melanoma, hepatoma, colon 26, mammary carcinoma C_3H or RIII), and leukemias (P388, L1210, AKR, C-1498) are useful routine tumors for the screening of new drugs, but grafted tumors are discredited by many scientists, who argue that they lack therapeutic predictability clinically. Are these methods helpful for the selection of an analogue? I would answer affirmatively if the assays are conducted methodically. It is necessary to consider the following points to differentiate the activities of drugs:

1. The schedule of the treatments (after grafting: early or postponed treatments).
2. The route of the treatments. With the anthracyclines, the I.V. route is recommended, but the other routes should be tested, even the oral route, since a few compounds are reported to be active orally, such as carminomycin or 4-demethoxy derivatives.[12]
3. The *therapeutic index* [ratio of the 50% lethal dose to the 50% activity dose (LD_{50}/AD_{50})] expresses the relationship between toxicity and antitumor activity. The comparison of the indexes of analogues should be assessed by convenient statistical methods.
4. The long survival of treated animals should be taken into account.
5. Using L1210 or glioma tumors grafted intracerebrally, the crossing of the meningeal blood barrier by new analogues should be studied. It is known that DNR and DOX do not.

The finding of systems in which the parent compounds are inactive would be useful. Combination chemotherapy may be considered and also "operational chemotherapy," such as surgical adjuvant chemotherapy.

INDUCED TUMORS

The grafted tumors are easy to manage for a screening program, but the need for new experimental animal models is obvious if we wish to approach the clinical situation (growth curve, biological markers, metastases). The induced tumors are proposed to answer this question, but they are more difficult to work with because of the long delay in tumor induction, individuality of the tumor evolution, and scattering of the resulting data. However, such tumor systems are recommended for the choice of a derivative. These tumors are induced by

1. Irradiation (a method using radioactive cerium chloride for induction of sarcomas and osteosarcomas in the rat is currently being evaluated at this Institute[16])
2. Oncogenic viruses
3. Chemicals (dimethylbenzanthracene, methylcholanthrene, benzpyrene)

The use of such a tumor system is explained in detail by M Denechaud *et al.* in Chapter 2.

SPONTANEOUS TUMORS

With spontaneous tumors, we are apparently closer to the human situation, for example, AKR leukemia and RIII mammary carcinoma. The facilities of large breeding units are necessary for working on such tumors in experimental chemotherapy.

The collaboration of veterinary surgeons interested in experimental chemotherapy is very useful because oncogenesis in domestic animals is frequently encountered, for example, mammary carcinomas, leukemias, and osteosarcomas in dogs and cats.

HETEROGRAFTED HUMAN TUMORS

Human tumors (lung, colon, breast) may be grafted

1. On egg chorioallantoic membrane
2. In the cheek pouch of the hamster
3. Under the renal capsule (mice and rats)
4. In immunodepressed animals
5. In nude mice[17]

The study of DOX analogues against human colon carcinoma xenografts has given interesting results, showing that new derivatives could give varying action against different human tumors.[18,19]

Toxicological Studies

Comparative toxicological studies are needed for the selection of analogues. To fulfill this important program at an acceptable level, time, space, research, and money are required. As a guideline, it is advisable to refer to reliable articles devoted to the comparative toxicity of anticancer agents.[20]

Different species should be used, such as mice, rats, rabbits, hamsters, cats, dogs, and monkeys.

LD_{50}, LD_{10}, and maximum tolerated dose should be carefully determined and statistically analyzed.

The toxicities for the following organs and tissues should be studied: (1) blood, bone marrow, (colony-forming unit-spleen and colony-forming unit-culture); (2) liver (SGOT, SGPT); (3) gastrointestinal tract; (4) kidney (blood urea nitrogen, creatinine); (5) central nervous system; (6) genital glands; (7) respiratory tract; (8) skin (alopecia in hamster and cats[21]); and last, but not least, (9) cardiotoxicity.

The following compounds have a detoxifying action: ICRF-159,[22] DNA complexes,[23] liposomes,[24] coenzyme Q10,[25,26] and superoxide dismutase (S.O.D.).

Mutagenic, Teratogenic, and Carcinogenic Activities

The genetic toxicology, embryotoxicity, and carcinogenic potential of analogues should be evaluated and compared.

MUTAGENIC ACTIVITY

The mutagenic activity of anthracycline derivatives may be studied using various tests, for example:

1. Chromosome aberrations[27-29]
2. Sister chromatid exchanges
3. Level of DNA repair
4. Microorganic tests (Salmonella typhimurium or Ames test, Escherichia coli, Neurospora crassa, Saccharomyces cerevisiae)
5. Chinese hamster cell mutation test

A dose-dependent activity should be established. In these tests, DNR and DOX are usually found to be active.[30]

In the chromosome aberration test, carminomycin is more potent than DNR.[31] DNR and DOX are nearly as active as other strong mutagens in V 79 hamster cells.

Inactive antitumor analogues such as 1'-epiadriamycin did not show mutagenic activity in this system. 4'-Epiadriamycin and 4-demethoxyadriamycin are potent antitumor compounds and also strong mutagens in the chromosome test.[32]

With the Ames technique, using the more sensitive TA 98 his⁻ strain (frameshift mutation), we have studied the activity of various analogues: the least active are DNR and rubicyclamin; detorubicin is less active than DOX. The absence of mutagenic activity in the Ames test of aclacinomycin A should be noted.[33]

TERATOGENIC ACTIVITY

We have found that DNR is teratogenic in the chick embryo, but not in the rabbit under our experimental conditions.

Thompson et al.[34,35] have demonstrated the embryotoxic and teratogenic properties of DOX and DNR, administered I.P. in rats (on a mg/kg basis, DOX was a more potent teratogen), but none of the drugs were clearly teratogenic in the rabbit by I.V. administration.

In mice, carminomycin is more embryo-toxic than the other parent anthracyclines and is also teratogenic, but the pattern of malformations induced is different from those seen in rat fetuses exposed to DOX or DNR.[36]

CARCINOGENIC ACTIVITY

In cell cultures (Fischer rat embryo cell system), DOX acts as a transforming agent.[37]

In female rats, treated intravenously with a single high dose of anthracycline, a high incidence of mammary tumors was observed, mostly adenocarcinomas with DNR and fibroadenomas with DOX.[38,39] In rats again, renal tumors were observed following a single intravenous injection of DNR.[40]

Pharmacokinetic studies

IN VIVO

The achievements of pharmacokinetic studies of anthracyclines may be very helpful in better understanding the biological properties and activity spectrum of analogues in the laboratory and clinically. The results obtained during the study of organ distribution, metabolites, and excretion may explain and possibly predict the biological and clinical differences between analogues.

To perform such a comparative program, it is necessary to use reliable techniques such as chromatography and fluorometry, principally high-pressure liquid chromatography,[41-43] isotopic techniques ([3]H- and ^{14}C-labeled drugs, autoradiography), radioimmunoassay dosage,[44] and combined gas chromatography–mass spectrometry.[45]

We have the most extensive data at our disposal concerning DNR and DOX. In animals (mice, hamsters, and rats), differences in distribution and metabolism are reported with increased uptake of DOX and greater excretion of DNR.[46,47] Further comparative studies have been performed

with DNR and rubidazone,[48] and with DNR, DOX, and detorubicin,[49,50] which showed significant differences in tissue distribution and metabolites.

A relationship between cardiac toxicity and anthracycline distribution in the heart has been studied.[51] Differences between heart fixation of DNR and rubidazone have been observed.[48]

The major metabolites of DNR and DOX are daunorubicinol (13-hydroxy-DNR) and adriamycinol (13-hydroxy-DOX). DNR-ol is produced in larger proportion than DOX-ol, DNR is a preferable substrate for the cytoplasmic aldo-keto reductase.[52]

In animals and *in vitro* (tissue homogenates), DNR-ol or DOX-ol are transformed to hydrolytic products, the respective aglycones.[52]

STUDY AT THE CELLULAR AND MOLECULAR LEVEL

Pharmacological and pharmacokinetic studies at the cell level (cell uptake, efflux, cell distribution) help to understand differences in biological activities of analogues.

Anthracyclines are *mitostatic agents* that block the cell cycle in late S and G_2 phase.[53] *Cell uptake and localization* of these drugs are studied by fluorescence microscopy and by cell fractionation.[54] Differences in localization are observed under fluorescence microscopy in connection with the chemistry of the analogue under test, e.g., DNR and DOX are localized mainly in the cell nuclei, whereas AD-32 and aclacinomycin A are localized mainly in the cytoplasm.[55] It has been ascertained that DNR is more lysosomotropic than DOX, when using cell fractionation.

Action on nucleic acid synthesis

All the anthracycline derivatives inhibit both thymidine incorporation into DNA and uridine incorporation into RNA.[56] The anthracyclines may be divided into two groups on the basis of their activity on DNA and RNA synthesis[57]:

Group 1: Compounds that inhibit DNA and RNA synthesis at approximately comparable concentrations (DNR, DOX, carminomycin, pyrromycin).

Group 2: Compounds that inhibit whole-RNA synthesis at six- to sevenfold lower concentrations than those required to inhibit DNA synthesis, and nucleolar RNA synthesis at 170- to 1250-fold lower concentrations than necessary to inhibit DNA synthesis (compounds with di- or trisaccharides in the molecule, such as aclacinomycin A, marcellomycin, and musettamycin).

The study of activity on the reproduction of RNA and DNA viruses may give supplementary information on the comparative mode of action of new analogues.[58]

New anthracycline drugs should be studied in greater depth in order to understand the molecular mechanism of action, that is, the degree of DNA intercalating potency (affinity for DNA), and the importance of free radical formation responsible for toxicity and pharmaceutic action.[59]

Conclusions

The differences in activity observed in the study of anthracycline analogues are the result of numerous factors, for example:

1. Macromolecular binding, DNA damage
2. Membrane transport, drug retention
3. Interaction with subcellular target organs
4. Free radical formation
5. Metabolites
6. Immunopharmacology

The aim of research in this field is to gather "data on structure–activity relationship which would correlate experimental results with clinical predictability."[60]

REFERENCES

1. Dubost M, Ganter P, Maral R, Ninet L, Pinnert S, Preud'homme J, Werner GH: Un nouvel antibiotique à propriétés cytostatiques: La rubidomycine. *CR Acad Sci [D] (Paris)* 257: 1813, 1963.
2. Arcamone F, Cassinelli G, Fantini G, Grein A, Orezzi P, Pol C, Spalla C: Adriamycin, 14-hydroxydaunomycin, a new antitumor antiobiotic from *S. peucetius* var. *caesius*. *Biotechnol Bioeng* 11: 1101, 1969.
3. Maral R, Ponsinet G, Jolles G: Etude de l'activité antitumorale expérimentale d'un nouvel antiobiotique semi-synthétique: La rubidazone (22 050 RP). *CR Acad Sci [D] (Paris)* 275: 301, 1972.
4. Maral R, Ducep JB, Farge D, Ponsinet G, Reisdorf D: Préparation et activité antitumorale expérimentale d'un nouvel antibiotique semi-synthétique: La diéthoxyacétoxy-14 daunorubicine (33921 RP). *CR Acad Sci [D] (Paris)* 286: 443, 1978.
5. Di Marco A, Casazza AM, Gambetta R, *et al.*: Relationship between activity and aminosugar stereochemistry of daunorubicin and adriamycin derivatives. *Cancer Res* 36: 1962, 1976.
6. Israel M, Modest EJ, Frei E III: N-Trifluoroacetyladriamycin-14-valerate, an analog with greater experimental antitumor activity and less toxicity than adriamycin. *Cancer Res* 35: 1365, 1975.
7. Oki T, Matsuzawa Y, Yoshimoto A, Numata K, Kitamura I, Hori S, Takamatsu A, Umezawa H, Ishizuka M, Naganawa H, Suda H, Hamada M, Takeuchi T: New antitumor antibiotics, aclacinomycins A and B. *J Antibiot (Tokyo)* 28 (10): 830–836, 1975.
8. Umezawa H, Takahashi Y, Kinoshita M, Naganawa H, Masuda T, Ishizuka M, Tatsuta K, Takeuchi T: Tetrahydropyranyl derivatives of daunomycin and adriamycin. *J Antibiot (Tokyo)* 32: 1082, 1979.
9. Gause GF, Brazhnikova MG, Shorin VA: *Cancer Chemother Rep* 58 (2): 255, 1974.
10. Jolles G, Maral R, Messer M, Ponsinet G: Antitumor activity of daunorubicin derivatives. *Chemotherapy* 8: 237, 1976.
11. Henry DW: Structure-activity relationship among daunorubicin and adriamycin analogs. *Cancer Treat Rep* 63(5): 845, 1979.
12. Casazza AM: Experimental evaluation of anthracycline analogs. *Cancer Treat Rep* 63(5): 835, 1979.
13. Chabbert Y, Vial H: *Exp Cell Res* 22: 64, 1961.
14. Salmon SE, Hamburger AW, Soehnlen B, Durie BG, Alberts DS, Moon TE: Quantitation of differential sensitivity of human tumor stem cells to anticancer drugs. *N Engl J Med* 298: 1321, 1978.
15. Lotem J, Sachs L: Potential pre-screening for therapeutic agents that induce differentiation in human myeloid leukemia cells. *Int J Cancer* 25: 561, 1980.
16. Klein B, Pals S, Masse R, Lafuma J, Morin M, Binart N, Jasmin JR, Jasmin C: Studies of bone and soft-tissue tumours induced in rats with radioactive cerium chloride. *Int J Cancer* 20: 112, 1977.
17. Fodstad O, Aass N, Pihl A: Response to chemotherapy of human malignant melanoma xenografts in athymic nude mice. *Int J Cancer* 25: 453, 1980.
18. Giuliani FC, Kaplan NO, Coirin AK, Howell SB: Screening of new doxorubicin analogs with activity against human colon carcinoma xenografts. *Proc Am Assoc Cancer Res* 21 (1090): 272, 1980.
19. Giuliani FC, Kaplan NO: New doxorubicin ana-

logs active against doxorubicin-resistant colon tumor xenografts in the nude mouse. *Cancer Res 40: 4682, 1980*.

20. Freireich EJ, Gehan EA, Rall DP, Schmidt LH, Skipper HE: Quantitative comparison of toxicity of anticancer agents in mouse, rat, hamster, dog, monkey and man. *Cancer Chemother Rep 50: 219, 1966*.

21. Henness AM, Theilen GH, Lewis JP: Clinical investigation of daunorubicin, doxorubicin and 6-thioguanine in normal cats. *Am J Vet Res 38 (4): 521, 1977*.

22. Herman EH, Mhatre RM, Lee IP, Waravdekar VS: Prevention of the cardiotoxic effects of adriamycin and daunomycin in the isolated dog heart. *Proc Soc Exp Bio Med 140 (1): 234, 1972*.

23. Trouet A, Deprez-De Campeneere, D, De Duve C: Chemotherapy through lysosomes with a DNA-daunorubicin complex. *Nature [New Biol] 239:110, 1972*.

24. Juliano RL, Stamp D, McCullough N: Pharmacokinetics of liposome-encapsulated antitumor drugs and implication for therapy. *Ann NY Acad Sci 308: 411, 1978*.

25. Kishi T, Watanabe T, Folkers K: Bioenergetics in clinical medicine: Prevention by forms of coenzyme Q of the inhibition by adriamycin of coenzyme Q10—Enzymes in mitochondria of the myo-cardium. *Proc Nat Acad Sci USA 73(12): 4653, 1976*.

26. Shaeffer J, El-Mahdi AM, Nichols RK: Coenzyme Q10 and Adriamycin toxicity in mice. *Res Commun Chem Pathol Pharmacol 29(2): 309, 1980*.

27. De Grouchy J, De Nava C: Effets cytogénétiques de la rubidomycine. *Ann Genet (Paris) 11: 39, 1968*.

28. Kusyk C, Hsu TC: Adriamycin-induced chromosome damage: Elevated frequencies of isochromatide aberration in G_2 and S phases. *Experientia 32(12): 1513, 1976*.

29. Vig BK: Chromosome aberration induced in human leukocytes by the antileukemic antibiotic adriamycin. *Cancer Res 31(1): 32, 1971*.

30. Vig BK: Mutagenic effects of some anticancer antibiotics. *Cancer Chemother Pharmacol 3: 143, 1979*.

31. Kurlov OV, Koifman EK, Golber ED: Comparative cytogenic effect of carminomycin and rubomycin antitumor antibiotics. *Antibiotiki 23(6): 537, 1978*.

32. Marquardt H, Marquardt H: Induction of malignant transformation and mutagenesis in cell cultures by cancer chemotherapeutic agents. *Cancer 40(Suppl 4): 1930, 1977*.

33. Sugimura T, Umezawa K, Matsushima T, Sawamura M, Seino Y, Yahagi T, Nagao M: Mutagenicity of cancer drugs, prediction of the risk of a 2nd tumor and use of the mutation test for monitoring improvement of drugs. *Adv Cancer Chemother 8: 283, 1978*.

34. Thompson DJ, Molello JA, Le Beau JE: Differential sensitivity of the rat and the rabbit to the teratogenic and embryotoxic effects of eleven antineoplastic drugs. *Toxicol Appl Pharmacol 45(1): 353, 1978*.

35. Thompson DJ, Molello JA, Strebing RJ, Dyke IL: Teratogenicity of adriamycin and daunomycin in the rat and rabbit. *Teratology 17(2): 151, 1978*.

36. Damjanov I, Celluzzi A: Embryotoxicity and teratogenicity of the anthracycline antibiotic carminomycin in mice. *Res Commun Chem Pathol Pharmacol 28(3): 497, 1980*.

37. Price PJ, Suk WA, Skeen PC, Chirigos MA, Huebner RJ: Transforming potential of the anticancer drug, adriamycin. *Science 187: 1200, 1975*.

38. Bertazzoli C, Chieli T, Solcia E: Different incidence of breast carcinomas or fibroadenomas in daunomycin or adriamycin treated rats. *Experientia 27(10): 1209, 1971*.

39. Solcia E, Ballerini L, Bellini O, Sala L, Bertazzoli C: Mammary tumors induced in rats by adriamycin and daunorubicin. *Cancer Res 38(5): 1444, 1978*.

40. Sternberg SS, Philips FS, Cronin AP: Renal tumors and other lesions in rats following a single intravenous injection of daunomycin. *Cancer Res 32: 1029, 1972*.

41. Strauss JF, Kitchens RL, Patrizi VW, Frenkel E: Extraction and quantification of daunomycin and doxorubicin in tissues. *J Chromatogr 221: 139, 1980*.

42. Robert J: Extraction of anthracyclines from biological fluids for H.P.L.C. evaluation. *J Liq Chromatogr 3(10): 1561, 1980*.

43. Andrews PA, Brenner DE, Chou FTE, Kubo H, Bachur N: Facile and definitive determination of human adriamycin and daunorubicin metabolites by high-pressure liquid chromatography. *Drug Metab Dispos 8(3): 152, 1980*.

44. Van Vunakis H, Langone JJ, Riceberg LJ: Radioimmunoassays for adriamycin and daunomycin. *Cancer Res 34: 2546, 1974*.

45. Roboz J: *Mass Spectrometry in Cancer Research*. Academic Press, New York, 1978.

46. Di Fronzo G, Gambetta RA, Lenaz L: Distribution and metabolism of adriamycin in mice, comparison with daunorubicin. *Rev Eur Etud Clin Biol 16: 572, 1971*.

47. Yesair DW, Schwartzbach E, Shuck D, Denine EP, Asbell MA: Comparative pharmacokinetics of daunomycin and adriamycin in several animal species. *Cancer Res 32(6): 1177, 1972*.

48. Baurain R, Deprez-De Campeneere D, Trouet A: Distribution and metabolism of rubidazone and daunorubicin in mice. A comparative study. *Cancer Chemother Pharmacol 2(1): 37, 1979*.

49. Deprez-De Campeneere D, Baurain R, Trouet A: Pharmacokinetic, toxicologic and chemotherapeutic properties of detorubicin in mice: A comparative study with daunorubicin and doxorubicin. *Cancer Treat Rep 63: 861, 1979*.

50. Mhatre RM, Herman EH, Waravdekar VS, Lee IP: Distribution and metabolism of daunomycin, adriamycin and N-acetyldaunomycin in the Syrian golden hamster. *Biochem Med 6(5): 445, 1972*.

51. Bachur NR, Egorin MJ, Hildebrand RC: Daunorubicin and adriamycin metabolism in the golden syrian hamster. *Biochem Med 8(3): 352, 1973*.

52. Bachur NR: Adriamycin-daunorubicin cellular

pharmacokinetics. *Biochem Pharmacol 2 (Suppl):* *207, 1974.*

53. Raju MR, Johnson TS, Tokita N, Gillette EL: Flow cytometric applications to tumour biology: Prospects and pitfalls. *Br J Cancer Suppl 4: 171, 1980.*

54. Tulkens P, Beaufay H, Trouet A: Analytical fractionation of homogenates from cultivated rat embryo fibroblasts. *J Cell Biol 63: 383, 1974.*

55. Egorin MJ, Clawson RE, Cohen JL, Ross LA, Bachur NR: Cytofluorescence localization of anthracycline antibiotics. *Cancer Res 40: 4669, 1980.*

56. Meriwether WD, Bachur NR: Inhibition of DNA and RNA metabolism by daunorubicin and adriamycin in L1210 mouse leukemia. *Cancer Res* *32: 1137, 1972.*

57. Crooke ST, Duvernay VH, Galvan L, Prestayko AW: Structure–activity relationships of anthracyclines relative to effects on macromolecular syntheses. *Mol Pharmacol 14: 290, 1978.*

58. Papas TS, Schafer MP: The inhibition of Rauscher leukemia virus and avian myeloblastosis virus DNA polymerase by anthracycline compounds. *Ann NY Acad Sci 284: 566, 1977.*

59. Bachur NR, Gordon SL, Gee MV: A general mechanism for microsomal activation of quinone anticancer agents to free radicals. *Cancer Res 38(6): 1745, 1978.*

60. Carter SK: Anthracycline analogs: Reassessments and prospects. *Cancer Treat Rep 63(5): 935, 1979.*

CHAPTER 2

Use of Induced Tumors in Mice

M. Denechaud,[a] M. Laval,[a] and C. Jasmin[b]

The antitumoral effectiveness of molecules has usually been studied on transplanted tumors, which grow uniformly and rapidly, unlike human tumors.

To approximate clinical conditions, we produced slow-growing experimental tumors. Growth and cellular kinetic parameters for solid autochthonous chemically induced tumors in mice were statistically defined.[1-3]

The study was in two parts:

1. Comparison of the reaction of autochthonous soft tissue tumors and of transplanted tumors to various injections of adriamycin (ADM). The growth kinetics of our experimental model were found to be similar to those of human tumors.
2. Determination of the extent to which results obtained with experimental tumors could be extrapolated to human tumors by testing the toxicity and the antitumoral effectiveness of four anthracyclines: ADM, AD-143, 4'-epi-ADM, and detorubicin (DTR).

Material and Methods

EXPERIMENTAL MODELS

Autochthonous tumors were induced on 8 week-old Swiss male mice by injec-

[a]Laboratoire de Physique Nucléaire Appliquée et Radiobiologie Université de Bordeaux II, Bordeaux Cédex, France

[b]Institut de Cancérologie et d'Immunogénétique (I.C.I.G.) Hôpital Universitaire Paul-Brousse, Villejuif Cédex, France

tions of dimethylbenzanthracene (DMBA). A connective tissue tumor is obtained by one I.M. injection in the left posterior thigh muscle of 500 μg DMBA dissolved in 0.1 ml sesame oil.

The tumors used for transplantation were radioinduced carcinomas in line XVII male and female mice.

The four anthracyclines studied were ADM, 4'-epi-ADM, AD-143, and DTR. ADM and 4'-epi-ADM were dissolved in sterile water, AD-143 and DTR in phosphate buffer (pH 7.4 and 6.8, respectively). Each of these was injected I.V. into the mouse's tail at the following doses: 7.5 mg/kg for ADM, 75 mg/kg for AD-143, 1.2 mg/kg for 4'-epi-ADM, and 7.5 mg/kg for DTR. The ratio values of ADM per molecule are 1, 10, 0.2, 1.

PROTOCOLS

Mice were injected when their tumors reached a mean volume of 1.8 cm³. Molecules were injected I.V. in a 0.1–0.2 ml volume. I.P. injections were used when the edemal state of the tail did not allow I.V. injections.

KINETIC TUMOR PARAMETERS

The various parameters studied were as follows:

1. Growth delay: τ (the delay required for the tumor to regain its volume at the time of injection)
2. Therapeutic efficiency: η (the percentage of tumor reduction $\eta = 1 - V_{min}/V_{inj}$)
3. Survival delay after induction: SD_1, or after apparition: SD_2
4. Doubling times: DT_0 before treatment,

11

DT_1 when growth resumes after treatment

$$\text{Toxicity index } \beta = \frac{\Sigma M_i \times N_i}{\Sigma M_i}$$

where M_i = the number of mice that died after the ith injection, and N_i is the number of injections ($i = 1 \ldots 5$).

Results

COMPARISON OF AUTOCHTHONOUS AND TRANSPLANTED TUMORS

Transplanted tumors showed a rate of growth significantly faster than that of autochthonous tumors. Their volume was 1 cm³ 17 days after transplantation, with DT = 3 days and SD_1 = 32 (30–35) days, whereas autochthonous tumors reached a volume of 1 cm³ 124 days after initiation with DT = 5 days and SD_1 = 166 (158–176) days.

For these two tumor types, the volume reduction percentage τ increased with the number of injections N. After three ADM injections, $\eta \geqslant 50\%$ in 100% of transplanted tumors but in only 8% of autochthonous tumors. Thus, N was positively and significantly correlated with τ and SD. This was also the case between SD on the one hand, and τ and η on the other. The DT for tumor growth after treatment (DT_1) were not significantly different from those preceding the treatment (DT_0).

ANTITUMOR ACTION OF FOUR ANTHRACYCLINES

Molecules can be classified in increasing order of toxicity (as defined by β index): DTR (4.4), AD-143 (4.2), ADM (4.1), and 4'-epi-ADM (3.6). This classification coincides with SD_1 mean values (179, 177, 166, 170 days). Analysis of volume reduction rate after five injections shows that only ADM-treated mice have a reduction rate $\eta \geqslant 25\%$ (50% of these mice were concerned) (Fig. 1).

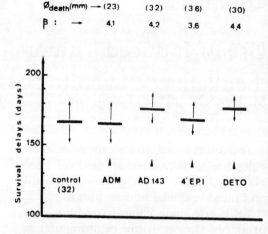

FIGURE 1.   Analysis of volume reduction rate after five injections of four anthracyclines.

ϕ death: Diameter at death
β Toxicity index

Conclusion

These preliminary results for four anthracyclines show that ADM used at the maximum tolerable dose is the most effective against soft tissue tumors.

The volume reduction rate observed after 4'-epi-ADM, DTR and AD-143 injections are lower than 25%.

4'-epi-ADM was injected at the maximum possible dose. It would be interesting to test the efficiency of DTR and of AD-143 by increasing the injected doses.

REFERENCES

1. Denechaud M, Ducassou D, Malaise E: Compared growth rate of chemically induced mice sarcoma and carcinoma. Ninth European Study Group Cell Proliferation, Paris, March 1978.
2. Denechaud M, Bioulac P, Ducassou D: Mathematical model of growth and cellular kinetics of autochthonous solid tumours with differentiated histology. Symposium on Cancer Modality Treatment and Cell Proliferation E.A.C.R., Budapest, October 1978.
3. Denechaud M, Ducassou D: Analyse statistique des cinétiques de croissance des épithéliomes et sarcomes chimio-induits chez la souris. *Bull Cancer (Paris) 67*(2): 161–165, 1980.

CHAPTER 3

In vitro Effect of Anthracyclines on Leukemic Progenitor Cells

J.P. Marie,[a] R. Zittoun,[a] and E. McCulloch[b]

It is clinically evident that the anthracyclines have a marked bone marrow toxicity. The inhibition of normal bone marrow colony-forming unit-granulo-monocytes (CFU-GM),[1,2] after their pre-incubation with an anthracycline, is the *in vitro* result of this toxicity.

The crucial point is to measure the *in vitro* antitumor activity of these drugs and to compare this activity to the CFU-GM toxicity.

The *in vitro* antitumor activity of anthracyclines has been tested on several animal lymphoma and leukemia continuous cell lines,[3,4] as well as on solid tumors.[5] These studies are useful for understanding the biochemical mechanisms of these drugs, but they do not help the clinician in the management of malignant disease.

It would be highly desirable to have a reliable test comparable to that used to assay sensitivities of bacteria to antibiotics. Such a system could be used to test the response of an individual patient's tumor cells to various drugs before starting chemotherapy.

Several investigators have examined the feasibility of *in vitro* predictions of clinical antitumor effect by the measurement of the incorporation of tritiated thymidine in fresh leukemic cells, before and after drug exposure,[6] with significant correlations between a high DNA synthesis inhibition produced by cytosine arabinoside and adriamycin and the attainment of complete remission induced by these drugs.[7] But these assays do not measure the ability of these drugs to kill the leukemic cells, since activation of these antitumor agents does not guarantee the presence of a critical drug sensitivity pathway, and inhibition of DNA synthesis is not necessarily lethal.

The recent development of leukemic myeloblast culture assays[1,8,9] permits study of the properties of the leukemic progenitor (CFU-L). Using such *in vitro* colony-forming assays for tumor stem cells, it has been further shown that *in vitro* chemotherapy sensitivity tests can predict the response to chemotherapy for tumors in man.[10,11]

Assay for Blast Cell Progenitor

Buick and McCulloch[8] have developed a blast culture assay in semisolid medium. Like early hematopoietic cells, the blast cell progenitor will form colonies in culture when provided with a semisolid support structure (methylcellulose) and suitable stimulation. The stimulator is contained in a medium conditioned by normal leukocytes in the presence of phytohemagglutinin (PHA-LCM). Under these conditions, the mononuclear cells from the blood of acute myeloblastic leukemia (AML) patients, depleted of T lymphocytes, will yield colonies containing more than 20 blast cells after 5–7 days of culture.[12] The proliferation basis of colony

[a]Service d'Hématologie de l'Hôtel-Dieu, Paris, France, and [b]Ontario Cancer Institute, Toronto, Canada

formation was demonstrated both by several examinations of cultures and by measuring a radiation sensitivity in the range characteristic of mammalian cell proliferation.[13] The validity of the assay is based on the morphological similarity between cells from blast colonies and those identified as blast in the blood of patients providing the culture, including the presence of a myeloid antigen (My-1) on the cell surface[14] and Auer bodies in the cultures. A firm link between blast colony formation and the leukemic process was demonstrated by observing chromosomal abnormalities, present in fresh preparations of marrow or blood within metaphases obtained from blast cell colonies. More recently, the validity of the assay has been confirmed by the finding that measurements obtained with the blast assay contribute to the variation between patients achieving remission and treatment failure.[15]

BLAST PROGENITOR PROPERTIES

The plating efficiency of blast cell populations varies between $1/10^4$ and $1/10^3$. These low values provided the first evidence that a progenitor existed among the blast cells, the majority of which were incapable of colony formation in response to PHA-LCM. By introducing an E-rosette depletion step, blast colony formation could be obtained even when recognizable blasts were few in the specimen, and T-cell colony formation was avoided almost entirely.[12]

Blast progenitor properties determined by manipulating the cells before, during, or after culture have proved more revealing.

Proliferative rate.

Blast populations were exposed briefly to either high specific activity tritiated thymidine or hydroxyurea, and then plated. Loss of colony formation after such exposure is considered to be the result of inactivation of cells in the DNA-synthetic phase of the cycle. For 15 AML patients, marked (about 50%) reduction in colony formation was found, indicating that blast progenitors were actively in cell cycle. The finding that blast progenitors are usually proliferatively active is important for the understanding of leukemic pathophysiology. It has particular significance for measurements of drug sensitivity in culture, since many drugs are phase or cycle specific.

Capacity for self-renewal.

The defining property of hematopoietic stem cells is the capacity for self-renewal.[15] Blast cell progenitors were shown to have this property by harvesting cells either from single colonies or pools of colonies and replating. Secondary colonies were observed with the same cultural requirement and cellular composition as the primary. These secondary colonies must have derived from new blast progenitors generated by the process of self-renewal during primary colonial growth. Renewal capacity was assessed quantitatively by measuring the plating efficiency of cell suspensions obtained from pooled colonies (secondary plating efficiency, or PE2). PE2 therefore represents a property of the population of blast progenitors.

Sensibility to Adriamycin.[2]

Adriamycin is a drug presently included in the remission induction protocol at the Princess Margaret Hospital (Toronto) and Hôtel-Dieu de Paris. Dose–response curves for killing effect of adriamycin on blast progenitors were obtained by exposing the cells to various drug concentrations (1–6 μg/ml = $2 \times 10^{-6}M$ to $10^{-5}M$) for 10 minutes, washing, and plating. These dose–response curves could be aproximated by a single negative exponential characterized by the drug dose that reduced survival to 10% of control (D_{10}); measurements of adriamycin D_{10} were found to be reproducible when the same sample was tested repeatedly, either when fresh or after cryopreservation. For 52 AML patients, the D_{10} adriamycin value has varied from very sensitive (<0.1 μg/ml or 2×10^{-7} M) to resistant (>5 μg/ml or 10^{-5} M). An example of such a study is provided in Figure 1, which displays adriamycin and daunorubicin dose–response curves for T lymphocyte colonies and granulopoietic progenitors were obtained with the same technique (10-minute exposure to anthracycline before plating). It is evident that, for both anthracyclines, blast cell colony formation was more sensitive to the chemotherapeutic agent than either of the normal populations chosen for comparison. The observation that anthracyclines, known to be useful in the treatment of leukemia, yield dose–response curves that differ for different cellular subpopulations provides initial support for the view that assay for blast cell progenitors may be of some value in assessing the drug sensitivities of subpopulations present in leukemia.

Comparison of drug sensitivity of blood and bone marrow leukemic progenitor cells.

We have compared adriamycin survival curves for blood and bone marrow blast cells progenitors in seven AML patients. The D_{10} (5×10^{-6} M) of the bone marrow leukemic progenitors is lower than the D_{10} of the blood leukemic progenitors (8×10^{-6} M), indicating that marrow leukemic cells seem to be more sensitive to adriamycin than blood leukemic cells.

CLINICAL CORRELATION OF DRUG SENSITIVITY

The *in vitro* sensitivity to adriamycin and cytosine arabinoside (Ara-C), used in the induction treatment, was tested as the parameter of predictive factor response to therapy, together with self-renewal (PE2). The results of a multiple regression analysis (logistic regression for 35 AML patients) are given in Table 1; the dependent

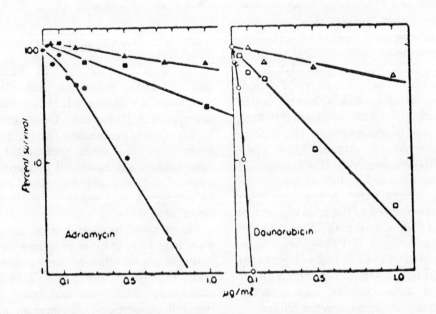

FIGURE 1.   Anthracycline survival curves for blast cell precursors (○●), CFU-C (□■), and T-cell colonies (△▲). (From *Cancer*, 42, 1978.)

TABLE 1. Logistic Regression Analysis of Association of Attributes with Remission Induction

Attribute	35 AML Patients, Percent of Variance (Cumulative)	p Value
PE2	14	0.025
Adriamycin D10	19	0.14
Ara-C D_{10}	20	0.45

variable was remission induction (1 = yes, 0 = no). PE2 was found to account at a significant level for 14% of the variance in occurrence of remission induction, and adriamycin sensitivity added only another 5%. The results provide support for the view that an aspect of the biological nature of AML clones (their self-renewal capacity measured by PE2) is more important in relation to remission induction than the response of the cells to the agents used in the treatment regimen.

Two other studies reported in 1980 demonstrate a significant correlation between the *in vitro* sensitivity to CFU-L to anthracyclines and other drugs.

Park et al.,[1,16] using a modified agar culture method with PHA-LCM that supports the growth of CFU-L from bone marrow AML, examined the *in vitro* response to chemotherapeutic agents of CFU-L in comparison with that of CFU-C (from hematologically normal patients) in 21 AML patients. The close survival experiments performed on CFU-C has permitted the empirical determination of the drug concentration that represents the threshold of survival of normal CFU-C (permitting 60–90% survival). It is $4 \times 10^{-7} M$ for adriamycin and $2 \times 10^{-7} M$ for rubidazone (1-hour exposure). A sensitive index (SI) was determined as the ratio of survival fraction of CFU-C to that of CFU-L. The SI was higher than 1 if CFU-L was more sensitive than CFU-C. A highly significant correlation was observed between high (or w) SI for anthracyclines and achievement of complete remission (or failure).

The mean of the SI for each drug used in the combination chemotherapy appears to be useful in predicting the response of the patient to chemotherapy.

Modification of the anthracycline time exposure (continuous exposure versus 1 hour) has not modified the correlation of SI with clinical response.[16]

Preisler,[9] using an agar culture assay with supernatant of continuous cell line as stimulator, tested the effect of daunorubicin (DNR) and Ara-C (drugs included in his AML induction protocol) on the AML blast colony formation.

The differences in CFU-L sensitivity to 0.1 μg/ml ($2 \times 10^{-7} M$) DNR, 1-hour exposure, between patients with drug-resistant disease and patients who entered into complete remission were significant ($p = 0.02$) for eight patients in complete remission ($44\% \pm 8\%$ of killed CFU-L) and six patients with resistant disease ($22\% \pm 4\%$).

The killing of CFU-L by DNR was more highly correlated with treatment outcome than was the effect of Ara-C on CFU-L, but the most sensitive test for recognizing leukemia that is sensitive or resistant to therapy with Ara-C and DNR has been exposure of leukemic cells to Ara-C and DNR simultaneously.

Conclusion

The work on blast cells in culture has matured to the point that progenitor cell properties are measured, rather than primary plating efficiencies. Drug sensitivity is one of these properties. The blast culture assay could be a useful tool to test the *in vitro* toxicity on blast cell progenitors of known and new anthracyclines and can help to select drug combinations in case of resistant disease.

But, finally, it should be remembered that drug sensitivity is only one factor in determining whether or not a patient will enter remission. The patient's biological characteristics and the leukemic progenitor cell properties (self-renewal, and so on) are also of importance in the outcome of remission induction therapy.

REFERENCES

1. Park CH, Amare M, Savin MA, Goodwin UN, Newcomb MM, Hoogstraten B: *Blood 55: 595, 1980*.
2. Buick RN, Messner HA, Till JE, McCulloch EA: *J Nat Cancer Inst 62: 249, 1979*.
3. Mantovani A: *Cancer Res 37: 815, 1977*.
4. Oki T, Takenchi T, Oka S, Umezama H: V US-Japan program review, San Francisco, 1979.
5. Morasca L, Fogarottaviano EG, Garattini S: *Eur J Cancer 12: 107, 1976*.
6. Zittoun R, Bouchard M, Faquet Danis J, Percie Du Sert M, Bousser J: *Cancer 35: 507, 1975*.
7. Dosik GM, Barlogie B, Johnston D, Millard D, Freireich EJ: *Eur J Cancer 17, 549, 1981*.
8. Buick RN, Till JE, McCulloch EA: *Lancet 1: 862, 1977*.
9. Preisler HD: *Blood 56: 361, 1980*.
10. Salmon SE, Hamburger AW, Soehnlen B, Durie BGM, Alberts DS, Moon TE: *N Engl J Med 298: 1321, 1978*.
11. Von Hoff DD, Page C, Harris G, Clark G, Cowan J, Coltman CA: *Proc Am Assoc Cancer Res 22: 610, 1981*.
12. Minden MD, Buick RN, McCulloch EA: *Blood 54: 186, 1979*.
13. Minden MD, Till JE, McCulloch EA: *Blood 52: 592, 1978*.
14. Marie JP, Izaguirre CA, Civin CI, Mirro J, McCulloch EA: *Blood 58:670, 1981*.
15. Buick RN, Minden MD, McCulloch EA: *Blood 54: 95, 1979*.
16. Park CH, Amare M, Wiernick PH, Maloney TR: *Proc Am Assoc Cancer Res 22: 603, 1981*.

CHAPTER 4

Immunological Effects of Aclacinomycin in Mice

S. Orbach-Arbouys, M. Ginsbourg, C. E. Andrade-Mena, and G. Mathé

Although it is difficult to determine which aspects of the immune response are of importance for cancer patients, the maintenance of a high capacity to respond is essential. The extensive use of clinical protocols associating immuno- and chemotherapy implies that the immunological machinery is not entirely annihilated by the administration of oncostatic drugs.

We addressed ourselves to the study of the modifications of the immunopotential after treatment by oncostatics, and our experimental protocol was designed to evaluate the immune responses remaining after drug administration, that is, the antigen was given after the drug.

Materials and Methods

Specific pathogen-free (C57B1/6 × DBA/2)F_1, (BDF$_1$), C57B1/6, or C$_3$H/He mice, 6- to 8-weeks old, were obtained from the breeding center of the Centre National de la Recherche Scientifique in Orléans-La Source, France. They were used within 2 weeks of arrival at the Institute.

The tumor C3-9, kindly obtained from Dr. G. Lespinats, I.R.S.C., Villejuif, is a methylcholanthrene-induced fibrosarcoma that was maintained by passage *in vivo*. For the experiments described, 10^5 cells that had been dissociated with trypsin were injected intradermally and the animals used when the tumor was larger than 1 cm in diameter.

Antibody-forming cells were assayed on day 6 after the intraperitoneal injection of 0.2 ml of 10% sheep red blood cell (SRBC) suspension. In order to test the T-independent antibody response, 3 μg of (TNP-LPS) in saline were injected intraperitoneally and the splenic antibody-forming cells of individual mice enumerated on day 3, using TNP-SRBC.

Delayed-type hypersensitivity reaction was elicited by painting the mice with a 3% (v/v) solution of oxazolone (BDH England) in acetone on day 0. On day +6 a challenge of 0.5% (v/v) oxazolone in an equal volume of acetone and olive oil was applied to one ear. Ear thickness was measured with a micrometer caliper 24 hours after the challenge. For each mouse, the difference between the treated ear and the control ear served as an indication of ear swelling and hence of the reaction to the hapten.

Results

The immune potential of aclacinomycin-treated mice was measured either by the plaque-forming cell (PFC) response to SRBC or by the delayed-type hypersensitivity reaction to oxazolone.

Increasing doses of aclacinomycin (1–8 mg/kg) were injected intraperitoneally 4 days before the T-dependent antigen, SRBC. The response of the mice injected with 4 mg/kg was signficiantly increased, whereas the other groups responded slightly less than the controls. Such an augmented response could still be observed 10–15 days after the drug injection. However, all subsequent tests were per-

Hôpital Universitaire Paul-Brousse, Institut de Cancérologie et d'Immunogénétique, Villejuif Cédex, France

formed 4 days after drug injection to minimize the possibility of an autorestoration occurring after cell destruction, similar to that often referred to as an "immunological rebound."

In contrast, the response to a T-independent antigen TNP-LPS was reduced in such animals. Furthermore, when aclacinomycin was injected *after* SRBC, the PFC response was decreased. The delayed-type hypersensitivity to oxazolone has been measured both in normal and in tumor-bearing animals. The response in the latter is much reduced. Both groups of responses are enhanced if aclacinomycin is injected 4 days before the immunization (Table 1).

Under the same conditions, aclacinomycin further enhanced the increased responses of adjuvant-treated mice, with BCG, 1 mg on day −14 or with azimexon on day −7 (Table 2).

The cellular drug-induced alterations were also studied, using cellular enzyme markers described as T-cell specific. The presence of acid phosphatase[1] and acid esterase has been described as specific for T cells and some of their subgroups.[2] The bone marrow cells were harvested from mice injected 3, 5, or 20 days before with a 4 mg/kg aclacinomycin. As early as day 3, we observed an increase in the number of myeloblasts and the appearance of lympho-

TABLE 2. Augmentation by Aclacinomycin of the Stimulating Effect of Azimexon on the Hypersensitivity to Oxazolone of Normal and Tumor-bearing Mice

Treatment	Ear Swelling (1/10 mm ± SD)	
	Normal Mice	Tumor-bearing Mice
Nil	9.8 ± 1.1	1.6 ± 1.6
Aclacinomycin day −4	20.0 ± 0.7	5.8 ± 1.3
Azimexon day −7	21.0 ± 0.7	9.0 ± 2.0
Azimexon day −7 + aclacinomycin day −4	25.2 ± 0.4	14.2 ± 1.6

cytes in which an acid phosphatase reactivity could be faintly seen, which may be interpreted as a maturation of bone marrow cells into T cells. The lack of acid esterase reactivity described as specific of T μ cells (T helper) suggests that the T cells are still immature. We see in Table 3 that the presence of acid phosphatase-positive lymphocytes increases with time.

Discussion

There are a few reports in the literature of increases of immune responses after the administration of oncostatic drugs, and it is very likely that many of these are not always immunosuppressive when examined in an appropriate way.

We have personally observed[3] that when methotrexate was injected 5 days before harvesting spleen cells for evaluation of their activity, the reaction *in vitro* to phytohemagglutinin or *in vivo* to histocompatibility antigens was increased. Cyclophosphamide at doses that do not affect B cells, and in consequence antibody production, also increased delayed hypersensitivity reactions; this has been interpreted as being due to the elimination of chemosensitive suppressor cells.[4]

Our results indicate that the overall immune reactivity of mice may be greatly enhanced by aclacinomycin treatment.

TABLE 1. Augmentation by Aclacinomycin of the Stimulating Effect of BCG on the Hypersensitivity to Oxazolone of Normal and Tumor-Bearing Mice

Treatment	Ear Swelling (1/10 mm ± SD)	
	Normal Mice	Tumor-bearing Mice
Nil	10.6 ± 1.3	1.8 ± 1.1
Aclacinomycin, day −4	13.6 ± 6.6	5.2 ± 0.4
BCG, 1 mg day −14	27.0 ± 2.8	7.6 ± 0.5
BCG, 1 mg day −14 + aclacinomycin, day −4	36.2 ± 1.1	11.2 ± 0.8

TABLE 3. Cellular Modifications in the Bone Marrow of Mice Injected with Aclacinomycin

		Bone Marrow Harvested on		
	Controls	Day +3	Day +6	Day +20
Myeloblasts	17	30 Some myelocytes	45 Promyelocytes Basophilic myelocytes	17
Erythroblasts	11	1	2	
Megacaryoblasts	+	+	+/++	+++
Polymorphonuclear	30	50	45	37
Lymphocytes	40	20	9	46
Acid phosphatase—positive[a]	0	0.02	0.9	15
Acid esterase—positive[a]	0	0	0	0

[a]"Dotlike" = T type.

Although additional experiments are required to define the precise mechanism of this phenomenon, we should stress the interest of the results obtained with the association of adjuvant aclacinomycin on the delayed-type hypersensitivity response, since the importance of the prognostic value of such a test in patients has been documented[5]: in inoperable lung cancer patients, the efficiency of chemotherapy in terms of regression and duration of remission is better in skin test-positive patients than in skin test-negative patients. When the cutaneous reactivity has been restored by BCG, the chemotherapy is then as active as in initially positive patients. Whatever may be the mechanism, the clinical implication might be of some importance.

Our results show also that, at least in mice, aclacinomycin does not depress the immune responses of tumor-bearing individuals, but actually enhances some immune functions.

The suggested cellular maturation we observed in the bone marrow of aclacinomycin-treated mice is of some interest, since some preliminary data suggest that the same holds true in man.

The acid phosphatase-positive cells are immature T cells or eventually T γ cells. The latter possibility cannot yet be formally excluded.

We are presently trying to find the mechanism of the observed enhancement, which may not be the same in tumor-bearing mice and in normal mice.

ACKNOWLEDGMENTS

This work was supported by contracts of the Délégation Générale à la Recherche Scientifique et Technique (78-2646) and of the Institut National de la Santé et de la Recherche Médicale (ATP 59-7891). C. E. Andrade-Mena received a fellowship from the Universidad de Guadalajara and Conacyt, Mexico.

The aclacinomycin used in this study was kindly donated by the Laboratoire Roger Bellon.

REFERENCES

1. Catovsky D: T-cell origin of acid phosphatase-positive lymphoblasts. Lancet 2: 327–328, 1975.
2. Grossi CE, Webb SR, Zicca A, Lydyard PM, Moretta L, Mingari MC, Cooper MD: Morphological and histochemical analysis of two human T-cell subpopulations bearing receptors for IgM and IgG. J Exp Med 147: 1405–1417, 1978.
3. Orbach-Arbouys S, Castes BM: Augmentation of immune responses after methotrexate administration. Immunology 36: 265, 1979.
4. Schwartz A, Askenase PW, Gershon RK: Regulation of delayed-type hypersensitivity reactions by cyclophosphamide sensitive T-cells. J Immunol 121: 1573, 1978.
5. Pouillart P, Schwarzenberg L, Huguenin P, Botto G, Gauthier H: Immune status, chemotherapy and lung cancer. Lancet : 5, 1976.

Part II

Cardiac Toxicity: Experimental

CHAPTER 5

Comparative Experimental Study and Evaluation of the Degree of Cardiotoxicity and Alopecia of Twelve Different Anthracyclines Using the Golden Hamster Model

D. Dantchev, M. Paintrand, C. Bourut, I. Pignot, R. Maral, and G. Mathé

Introduction

The cardiotoxicity, general toxicity, and alopecia of eight anthracyclines previously studied, adriamycin (ADM), detorubicin (DTR), daunorubicin (DNR), 4'-epiadriamycin (4'-epi-ADM), rubidazone (RBZ), aclacinomycin (ACM), N-trifluoroacetyladriamycin-14-valerate (AD-32), and tetrahydropyranyladriamycin (THP-ADM), are compared with the same toxic effects of four other anthracyclines recently studied, N-L-leucyldaunorubicin (L-DNR), carminomycin (CAM), rubicyclamin (RBC), and N-trifluoroacetyladriamycin-14-0-hemiadipate (AD-143), using our golden hamster model. This method enables detection of the degree of myocardial alterations, Grade 0 showing a normal electron microscopic (EM) structure; Grade 1, moderate toxic lesions; Grade 2, severe cardiac lesions; and Grade 3, very severe myocardial alterations.

According to the degree of their cardiotoxicity and the general toxicity and/or mortality, all the drugs studied are classified into three groups: 1) ADM, DNR, RBZ, and L-DNR, causing very severe cardiac lesions (Grade 2 and 3) and very high mortality; 2) 4'-epi-ADM, DTR, CAM, and RBC, causing severe cardiac alterations (Grade 1 and 1–2) and always very high mortality or general toxicity; and 3) ADM, AD-32, THP-ADM, and AD-143, causing lDM, and AD-143, causing less severe myocardial alterations (Grade 1 and 1–2) and extremely low mortality and general toxicity.

Cardiotoxicity and alopecia are the two main limiting factors for the use of anthracyclines in antitumor chemotherapy.[5,9,12,22] In clinical and experimental studies, many authors showed several biochemical changes and tissue alterations after treatment with these drugs, the binding of anthracyclines to nuclear and mitochondrial DNA being the main pathophysiological lesion, followed by an inhibition of RNA and protein synthesis.[1,2,4,10,13-15,18,19,21,23,24]

In a first trial, after administration of eight anthracyclines to golden hamsters, adriamycin (ADM), detorubicin (DTR), daunorubicin (DNR), 4'-epiadriamycin (4'-epi-ADM), rubidazone (RBZ), aclacinomycin A (ACM), N-trifluoroacetyladriamycin-14-valerate (AD-32), and tetrahydropyranyladriamycin (THP-ADM), we showed that electron microscopic (EM) findings of the myocardium and light microscopic (LM) findings of the skin could be predictive of the cardiotoxic effects and of the development of alopecia in man.[6-8]

Institut de Cancérologie et d'Immunogénétique, Hôpital Paul-Brousse, Villejuif Cédex, France

In a second trial, four other drugs, N-L-leucyldaunorubicin (L-DNR), carminomycin (CAM), rubicyclamin (RBC), and N-trifluoroacetyldaunorubicin-14-0-hemiadipate (AD-143) were studied, and in this chapter we report the results of the second trial, comparing them with those of the first trial.

This study confirms a low heart and skin toxicity, particularly for four new derivatives of ADM, ACM, AD-32, THP-ADM, and AD-143 that was reported in our preceding experimental study and also in some preliminary clinical observations.[3,6-8,16,20]

Materials and Methods

As was previously done,[6,7] 24 adult female golden hamsters were used for each drug, 12 of which served for evaluation of mortality. They received an I.P. administration three times a week for 4 weeks, a dose equivalent to three-fourths of the optimally oncostatic dose on murine L1210 leukemia when injected at days 1, 5, and 9 after tumor cell inoculation.[11] These doses are shown in Table 1.

Each week three hamsters for each drug and three controls were sacrificed and relevant tissues were quickly removed: the ventricular cross (apex) was immediately fixed for EM study in 5% cacodylate-buffered glutaraldehyde adjusted to pH 7.25, and the apex of the myocardium was minced under fixative into 1–2 mm³ blocks. The remainder of the heart and tissues, including lymph nodes, spleen, liver, kidneys, and skin, were collected for LM examination and fixed in 10% neutral-buffered formalin.

The blocks for EM study were postfixed in 2% osmium tetroxide, dehydrated in graded ethanols, transferred to propylene oxide, and embedded in Epon. Thin sections cut at 400–500 Å with a Porter-Bloom ultramicrotome were mounted on Form-var-coated 300-mesh copper grids, stained with uranyl acetate and lead citrate, and examined with a Jeol 100 C ASSID electron

TABLE 1.   Drug and Dose Used in Hamster

Drug	Dose Used in Hamster (mg/kg)
First Trial	
Adriamycin (ADM)	3
Daunorubicin (DNR)	3
Detorubicin (DTR)	3
4'-Epiadriamycin (4'-epi-ADM)	3
Rubidazone (RBZ)	9
Aclacinomycin (ACM)	6
N-Trifluoroacetyladriamycin-14-valerate (AD 32)	30
Tetrahydropyranyladriamycin (THP-ADM)	3
Second Trial	
Adriamycin (ADM)	3
N-L-leucyldaunorubicin (l-DNR)	6
Carminomycin (CAM)	0.15
Rubicyclamin (RBC)	7.5
N-Trifluoroacetyladriamycin-14-O-hemiadipate (AD 143)	60

microscope at 100 kV. For histopathological study the tissues were embedded in paraffin, sectioned at 6 μm, and stained with hematoxylin and eosin.

Results

MORTALITY AND GENERAL TOXIC OBSERVATIONS

Table 2 summarizes the number of surviving hamsters at the end of each week, and Figures 1 and 2 show the curves of mortality by toxicity in our two trials. It is evident that, in the first trial, mortality was very high for the first five drugs, ADM, DTR, DNR, 4'-epi-ADM, and RBZ, the majority of treated hamsters were dead between the first and third week, and all animals were dead before the end of the fourth week, with a loss of 30–40% of their weight and severe digestive troubles, particularly abundant diarrhea and great hair loss. Conversely, mortality was very low for the animals receiving ACM, AD-32,

TABLE 2. Mortality Due to Toxicity of Drug-Treated Animals (12 Animals per Group)

	No. of Animals Surviving at End of			
	1st Week	2nd Week	3rd Week	4th Week
First Trial				
ADM	12	7	0	0
DNR	12	7	0	0
DTR	12	7	4	0
4'-epi-ADM	12	12	7	0
RBZ	12	6	0	0
ACM	12	12	11	11
AD-32	12	12	12	11
THP-ADM	12	12	12	12
Second Trial				
ADM	12	4	0	0
L-DNR	12	8	0	0
CAM	12	11	4	0
RBC	11	11	9	7
AD-143	12	12	12	12

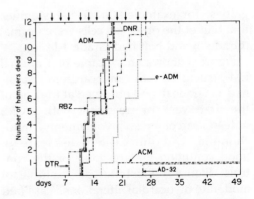

FIGURE 1. Curves of mortality in the first trial. Arrows indicate the I.P. administration of the drugs. There were no deaths with THP-ADM.

and THP-ADM, only 1 out of 12 ACM- and AD-32-treated hamsters died during the 4 weeks of treatment, and there were no deaths in the THP-ADM-treated animals. The ACM- and AD-32- and THP-ADM-treated hamsters preserved their good general status without loss of body weight, digestive troubles, or loss of hair.

In our second trial, mortality was also very high for the ADM-, L-DNR-, and CAM-treated hamsters, with no survivors at the end of the fourth week of treatment; mortality was a little lower for the RBC-treated animals, and some animals survived until the seventh week. Almost all animals treated with ADM and L-DNR had digestive troubles (diarrhea), a loss of body weight, and loss of hair. But these disorders were not evident in the CAM- and RBC-treated groups. All animals treated with AD-143 survived to the end of the fourth week of treatment and for many weeks later; their good general status was preserved without loss of body weight, digestive troubles, or loss of hair.

EM ALTERATIONS OF THE MYOCARDIUM

To establish a possible comparable appreciation of the degree of EM myocardial alterations, we used a grading system derived from that proposed by Billingham et al.[2] Grade 0 was used for a normal cardiac morphology; Grade 1 for the cases that contained some cells with moderate alterations; Grade 2 was assigned when more than 50% of myocardial cells showed severe alterations; and in Grade 3 the myocardium was diffusely affected by very severe cell alterations. We also used the intermediate grades of 0-1, 1-2, and 2-3, which indicate that about half the myocardial cells showed the morphological structure or changes of each of the two

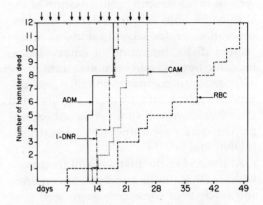

FIGURE 2. Curves of mortality in the second trial. The arrows indicate the I.P. administration of the drugs. There were no deaths with AD-143.

grades, for example, Grade 0-1 signifies that half of the observed cells were normal (Grade 0) and half had Grade 1 lesions.

Figure 3 shows an example of a normal EM structure of the myocardium, classified as Grade 0, and observed at the end of the first week of treatment with ACM; indeed, sarcomeres, myofilaments, mitochondria, and intercalated disks are in good condition, as are those of the controls. Figure 4 illustrates an example of moderate myocardial alterations, classified as Grade 1 and observed at the end of the first week of treatment with DTR, with a swelling of mitochondria and clearing of the matrices and lysis of the crests, separation and lysis of myofilaments, and disruption of Z-band registry. Figure 5 shows an example of severe myocardial alterations, classified as Grade 2, observed at the end of the first week of treatment with DTR, with swelling and clearing of mitochondria and lysis of their crests, clumping of the chromatin into electron-dense masses adjacent to the nuclear membrane and to the nucleoli, separation of the fascial adhesions of the intercalated disks, and formation of myelinic figures. Figure 6 shows an example of very severe myocardial alterations, classified as Grade 3, and observed at the end of the second week of treatment with DNR, with dilation of sarcoplasmic reticulum, separation and lysis of myofilaments, condensation of the chromatin into electron-dense masses, separation of fascial adhesions of intercalated disks, formation of empty space, myelinic figures, and vacuolization.

In order to compare mortality and degree of myocardial alterations at the end of each week, we will summarize our experimental data concerning two new drugs, L-DNR and AD-143.

At the end of the first week of treatment with L-DNR, mitochondria, sarcomeres, and nucleus of some cells were well preserved, but some other cells showed swelling of mitochondria with clearing of their matrices and lysis of the crests, dilation of

sarcoplasmic reticulum, and irregular nuclear membrane with clumping of the chromatin into electron-dense masses; these structures and alterations were classified as Grade 1. At the end of the second week, the myocardium showed the same alterations of the mitochondria, nuclei, and chromatin, separation and lysis of myofilaments with disruption of Z-band registry, and vacuolization; these lesions were classified as Grade 1-2. By this time four animals were dead. At the end of the third week of treatment, the myocardial alterations became very severe and were classified as Grade 2-3; at this time the remaining eight animals were also dead. Thus, according to these experimental data, L-DNR should be considered as a very cardiotoxic drug, giving a very severe general toxicity capable of killing all animals before the end of the experiment.

Generally at the end of the first week of treatment with AD-143, mitochondria, myofilaments, and nuclei were well preserved, but some cells showed alterations of their mitochondria, mild vacuolization, and formation of myelinic figures: these structures and lesions are classified as Grade 0-1. After 2 weeks treatment with AD-143, myocardial cells were mostly in good condition, but some cells showed alterations of the mitochondria, lysis of myofilaments, vacuolization, and formation of myelinic figures; these moderate lesions were classified as Grade 1. At the end of the third week of treatment, some cells were in good condition, whereas other cells showed swelling and clearing of mitochondria and lysis of the crests, and also separation of intercalated disks and clumping of the chromatin into electron-dense masses; these more severe alterations were classified as Grade 1-2. As shown in Table 1 and Figure 2, at this time of the treatment there were no dead animals. At the end of the fourth week of treatment with AD-143, some cells were well preserved, and others showed alterations of the mitochondria, separation of

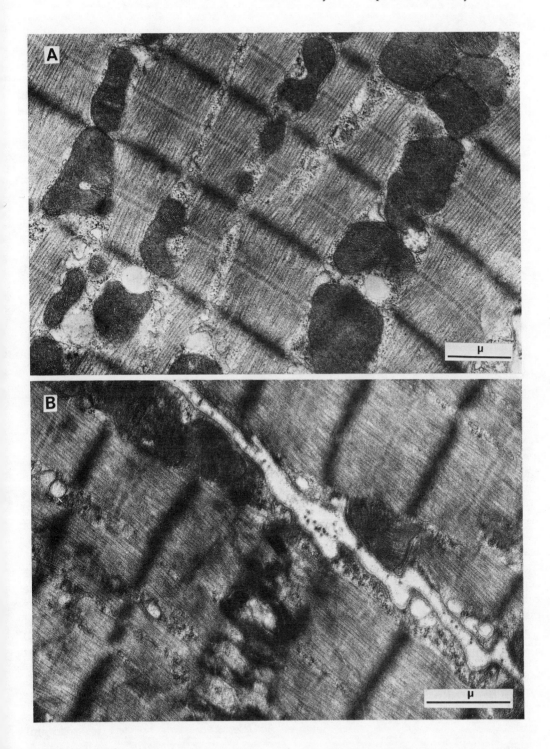

FIGURE 3. Myocardium from a golden hamster 7 days after treatment with ACM (6 mg/kg/injection I.P. three times a week) classified as Grade 0. Sarcomeres, mitochondria, myofilaments, and intercalated disks are in good condition, as are those of the controls.

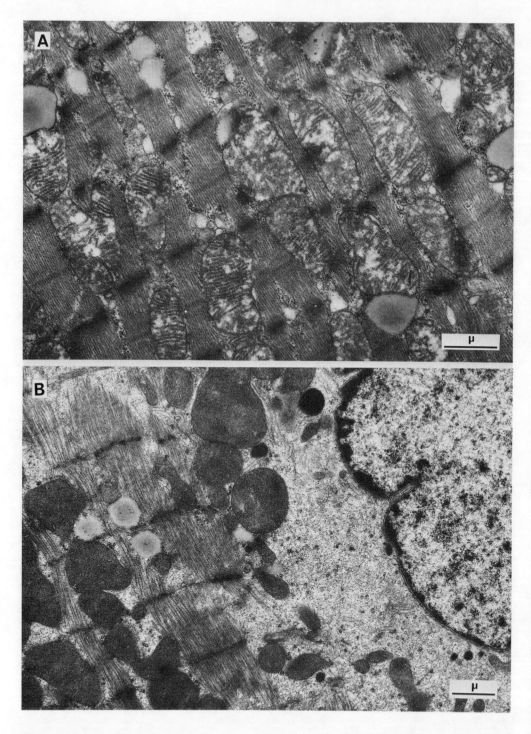

FIGURE 4. Myocardial alterations from a golden hamster 7 days after treatment with DTR (3 mg/kg/injection I.P. three times a week) classified as Grade 1, with swelling of mitochondria with clearing of their matrices and lysis of their crests, separation, loss of parallel orientation, and lysis of myofilaments with disruption of Z-band registry.

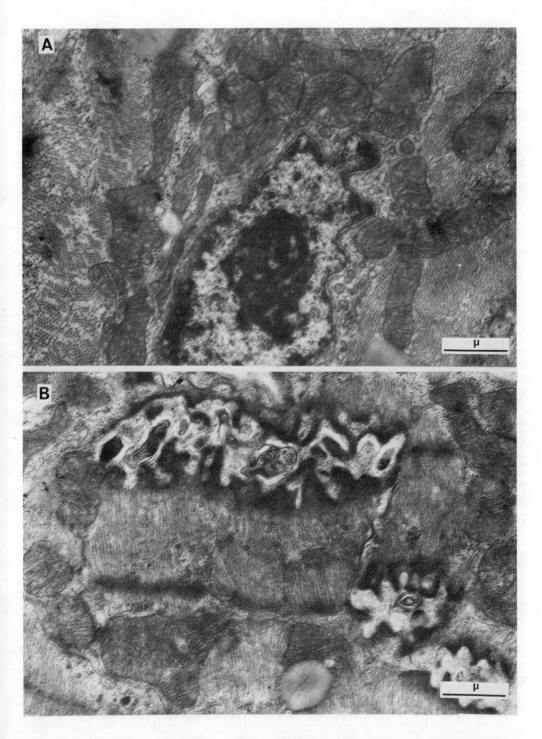

FIGURE 5. Myocardial alterations from a golden hamster 7 days after treatment with DNR (3 mg/kg/injection. I.P. three times a week) classified as Grade 2, with swelling and clearing of mitochondria with lysis of the crests, clumping of the chromatin into electron-dense masses, separation of the fascial adhesions of the intercalated disks, formation of myelinic figures.

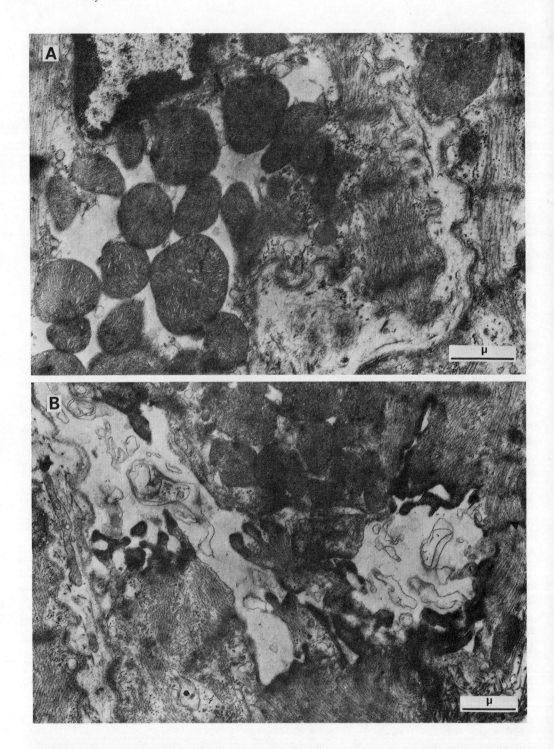

FIGURE 6. Myocardial alterations from a golden hamster 14 days after treatment with DNR (3 mg/kg-injection I.P. three times a week) classified as Grade 3, with dilation of sarcoplasmic reticulum, separation and lysis of myofilaments, condensation of the chromatin into electron-dense masses, separation of intercalated disks, formation of empty space and myelinic figures.

the intercalated disks, lysis of myofilaments, and formation of myelinic figures; these alterations were classified as Grade 1-2, and there were no animals dead, and all 12 hamsters were in good condition, without loss of body weight, digestive troubles, or loss of hair. Thus, AD-143 may be considered as not only giving low cardiotoxicity, but also causing low general toxicity; it is one of the least toxic anthracyclines that we studied.

Table 3 shows the degree of myocardial alterations at the end of each week of all drugs studied in our first and second trials according to our grading system and classification into three groups (see below).

Several observations can be drawn from this table. It is evident that all drugs studied are cardiotoxic; however, the degree of this cardiotoxicity, especially at the end of the first and second week of treatment, is different. According to the degree of the cardiotoxicity and the general toxicity, evaluated above all by the mortality, it is possible to classify all drugs studied into three groups: (1) ADM, DNR, RBZ, and L-DNR cause very severe myocardial alterations (Grades 2 and 3) and very high mortality; (2) 4'-epi-ADM, DTR, CAM, and RBC cause less severe myocardial alterations (Grades 1 and 1-2), but always very high mortality or general toxicity; and finally, (3) ACM, AD-32, THP-ADM, and AD-143 cause less severe myocardial alterations (Grades 1 and 1-2) and extremely low mortality and general toxicity. Almost all animals treated with these last four drugs survived, with very well-preserved general status, and 12 weeks after the treatment had been stopped the EM study of their myocardium revealed a recovery of myocardial alterations.

LESIONS OF THE SKIN

EM study of the myocardium enables detection of the degree of cardiotoxicity of different drugs, whereas the histopathologic study of the skin, at the end of each week of treatment, enables the evaluation

TABLE 3. Degree of Myocardial Electron-Microscopic Alterations at End of Each Week According to a Semiquantitative Grading System[a]

Classification of the 12 Drugs[b]	Degree of Myocardial Alterations at End of			
	1st Week	2nd Week	3rd Week	4th Week
First group				
ADM	1-2	2-3	2-3	
DNR	1-2	2-3		
4'-epi-ADM	1-2	2-3	2-3	
RBZ	1-2	2-3		
L-DNR	1	1-2	2-3	
Second group				
4'-epi-ADM	0-1	1-2	2	
DTR	0-1	1-2	2	
CAM	0-1	1-2	2	
RBC	0-1	1	1-2	1-2
Third group				
ACM	0-1	1	1-2	1-2
THP-ADM	0-1	1	1-2	1-2
AD-32	0-1	1-2	2	2
AD-143	0-1	1	1-2	2

[a]Grade 0: no pathologic alterations; Grade 1: moderate cell alterations; Grade 2: severe cell alterations; Grade 3: very severe cell alterations. Intermediate grades of 0-1, 1-2, and 2-3 indicate that about half of myocardial cells showed the morphological structure or alterations of each of the two grades.
[b]According to their degree of cardiotoxicity and general toxicity or mortality.

of degenerative lesions of the skin with alopecia caused by some drugs. However, it was sometimes difficult to distinguish typical lesions at the end of the first week, but, after the second week of treatment, particularly with ADM, DTR, DNR, 4'-epi-ADM, RBZ, and L-DNR, the skin showed very marked atrophy of all layers of the epidermis and a loss of hair, as shown in Figure 7. Conversely, the skin of animals treated with ACM, AD-32, THP-ADM, RBC, CAM, and AD-143 preserved normal histologic structure without loss of hair, even after 4 weeks of treatment, as shown in Figure 8.

Discussion

The clinical, as well as experimental ultrastructural and histopathological, studies of myocardial alterations induced by some

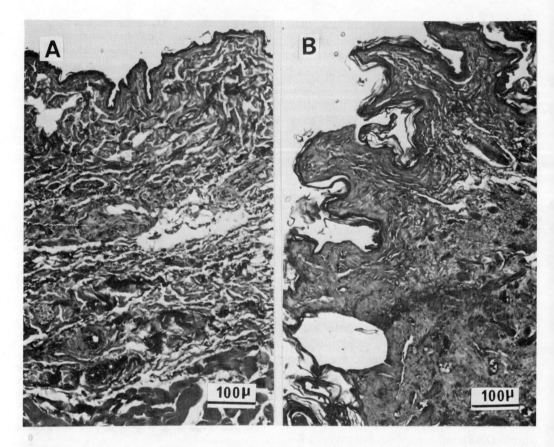

FIGURE 7. Histopathological alterations with the skin of a golden hamster after 3 weeks of treatment with ADM (A) and RBZ (B), showing atrophy of all layers of the epidermis and loss of the hair (alopecia).

anthracyclines, and especially by ADM, DNR, DTR, ADM-DNA, N-L-leucyladriamycin (L-ADM), and L-DNR, have been reported by several authors, who found numerous lesions of the myocardium which were similar to those in our published golden hamster model.[1,2,4,5,9,10,13,17-19,21-23]

The comparative study of mortality, EM alterations of the myocardium, the findings of general toxicity, and lesions of the skin, after administration of equivalent doses, enable several conclusions to be drawn concerning the toxic effects of the drugs studied in order to classify them and thus show the advantages and/or disadvantages of each one.

Because myocardial lesions were seen with all anthracycline drugs included in our first and second trials, it was of interest to find the degree of this cardiotoxicity, and also to evaluate the general toxicity of each drug under the same experimental conditions and at the same time.

These data are not sufficient in themselves to evaluate the toxic effects induced by the drugs studied. Careful microscopic analyses of many other organ samples, collected from sacrificed animals, must complete this study. Indeed, it has been shown by some authors that the toxic effects of anthracyclines cause severe troubles in many other organs and metabolites.[10] Nevertheless, our findings concerning cardiotoxicity, general toxicity,

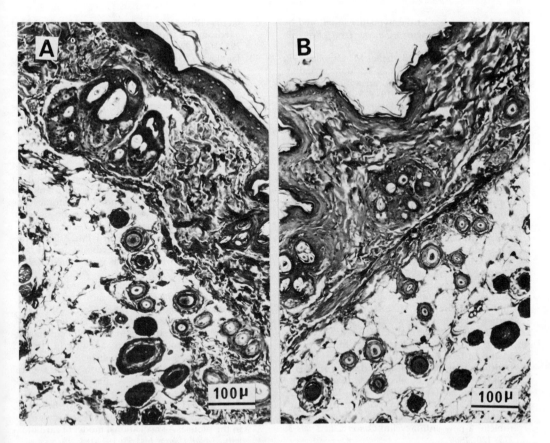

FIGURE 8. Histopathological alterations of the skin of a golden hamster after 4 weeks treatment with ACM (A) and AD-32 (B). Normal histological structure of epidermal cell layers and of the hair (no alopecia).

mortality, and lesions of the skin seem to be consistent with clinical data presently available with some of these drugs.[3,16,20]

One of the most interesting observations in our study is the demonstration of a possible recovery of myocardial lesions 2 and 3 months after the treatment had been stopped, especially in the animals treated with ACM, AD-32, and THP-ADM. The practical impact of these findings remains to be established in human beings.

In conclusion, after I.P. administration of 12 different anthracyclines to golden hamsters, the comparative study of mortality, the EM alterations of the myocardium, and the histopathologic lesions of the skin permit us to classify them into three groups, the last of which include the least toxic and especially the least cardiotoxic drugs: ACM, AD-32, THP-ADM, and AD-143. If, with this lower toxicity, the further clinical observations of these four drugs confirm a good antitumor activity, they will offer an important contribution to the chemotherapy of neoplasias.

REFERENCES

1. Benjamin RS, Mason YW, Billingham MD: Cardiac toxicity of adriamycin-DNA complex and rubidazone: Evaluation by electrocardiogram and endomyocardial biopsy. *Cancer Treat Rep* 62: 935–939, 1978.
2. Billingham ME, Mason JW, Bristow MR, Daniels

JR: Anthracycline cardiomyopathy monitored by morphologic changes. *Cancer Treat Rep 62: 865–872, 1978.*

3. Blum RH, Garnick MB, Israel M, Canellos GP, Henderson IG, Frei E III: *N*-Trifluoroacetyladriamycin-14-valerate (AD-32), an adriamycin analog. *Cancer Treat Rep 63: 919–923, 1979.*

4. Buja LM, Ferrans VJ, Mayer RJ, Roberts WC, Henderson ES: Cardiac ultrastructural changes induced by daunorubicin therapy. *Cancer 32: 771–788, 1973.*

5. Clarysse A, Kenis Y, Mathé G: *Cancer Chemotherapy. Its Role in the Treatment Strategy of Hematologic Malignancies and Solid Tumors.* Springer-Verlag, New York, 1976.

6. Dantchev D, Slioussartchouk V, Paintrand M, Bourut C, Hayat M, Mathé G. Electron microscopic studies of the heart and light microscopy of the skin after treatment of golden hamsters with adriamycin, detorubicin, AD-32 and aclacinomycin. *Cancer Treat Rep 63: 375–388, 1979.*

7. Dantchev D, Slioussartchouk V, Paintrand M, Bourut C, Hayat M, Mathé G. Ultrastructural study of the cardiotoxicity and light microscopic findings of the skin after treatment of golden hamsters with seven different anthracyclines. *Recent Results Cancer Res 74: 221–249, 1980.*

8. Dantchev D, Paintrand M, Hayat M, Bourut C, Mathé G: Low heart and skin toxicity of a tetrahydropyranyl derivative of adriamycin (THP-ADM) as observed by electron and light microscopy. *J Antibiot (Tokyo) 32(10): 1085–1086, 1979.*

9. EORTC Clinical Screening Group: Preliminary results of a Phase II trial on solid tumors of detorubicin, a new anthracyclin. *Cancer Clin Trials 3: 115–120, 1980.*

10. Ferrans VJ: Overview of cardiac pathology in relation to anthracycline cardiotoxicity *Cancer Treat Rep 62: 995–961, 1978.*

11. Freireich EJ, Gehan EA, Rall DP, Schnidt LM, Skipper HE: Quantitative comparison of toxicity of anticancer agents in mouse, rat, hamster, dog, monkey and man. *Cancer Chemother Rep 50: 219–245, 1966.*

12. Jacquillat C, Auclerc MF, Weil M, *et al.*: Clinical activity of detorubicin: A new anthracycline derivative. *Cancer Treat Rep 63: 889–893, 1979.*

13. Jaenke RS: An anthracycline antibiotic-induced cardiomyopathy in rabbits. *Lab Invest 30: 292–304, 1974.*

14. Jaenke RS, Deprez-De Campeneere D, Trouet A: Cardiotoxicity and comparative pharmacokinetics of six anthracyclines in the rabbit. *Cancer Res 40: 3530–3536, 1980.*

15. Lampidis TJ, Henderson IC, Mervyn I, Canellos GP: Structural and functional effects of adriamycin on cardiac cells *in vitro. Cancer Res 40: 3901–3909, 1980.*

16. Mathé G, Bayssas M, Gouveia J, Dantchev D, Ribaud P, Machover D, Misset JL, Schwarzenberg L, Jasmin C, Hayat M: Preliminary results of a phase II trial of aclacinomycin in acute leukemia and lymphosarcoma. An oncostatic anthracycline that is rarely cardiotoxic and induces no alopecia. *Cancer Chemother Pharmacol 1: 259–262, 1978.*

17. Mettler FP, Young DM, Ward JM: Adriamycin-induced cardiotoxicity (cardiomyopathy and congestive heart failure) in rats. *Cancer Res 37: 2705–2713, 1977.*

18. Olson HM, Capen CC: Subacute cardiotoxicity of adriamycin in the rat. Biochemical and ultrastructural investigations. *Lab Invest 37: 386–384, 1977.*

19. Olson HM, Young DM, Prieur DJ, Le Roy AF, Reagan RL: Electrolyte and morphologic alterations of myocardium in adriamycin treated rabbits. *Am J Pathol 77: 439–450, 1974.*

20. Ogawa M, Inagaki J, Horikoshi N, *et al.*: Clinical study of aclacinomycin A. *Cancer Treat Rep 63: 1979.*

21. Rosenoff SH, Olson HM, Young DM, Bostick F, Young RC: Adriamycin-induced cardiac damage in the mouse: A small animal model of cardiotoxicity. *J Natl Cancer Inst 55: 191–194, 1975.*

22. Trouet A, Sokal G: Clinical studies with daunorubicin-DNA and adriamycin-DNA complexes: A review. *Cancer Treat Rep 63: 895–898, 1979.*

23. Wakabayashi T, Oki T, Tone H, Hirano S, Omori K: A comparative electron microscopic study of aclacinomycin and adriamycin cardiotoxicities in rabbits and hamsters. *J Electron Microsc (Tokyo) 29(2): 106–118, 1980.*

24. Young, DM: Pathologic effects of adriamycin (NSC-123127) in experimental systems. *Cancer Chemother Rep 6: 159–175, 1975.*

CHAPTER 6

An *In Vitro* Model of Anthracycline Cardiopathogenesis

T. J. Lampidis

Function and Structure

Cardiac muscle cells are unique in that they maintain their ability to beat in culture for prolonged periods. In order to utilize the beating as a measure of physiological function we have constructed a closed microscopic stage that controls temperature and pH, two variables to which cardiac cell beating is particularly sensitive. An electronic monitoring system was developed to measure quantitatively and record beating patterns. The system consists of a video camera (RCA, model TC 1005) that transmits the image of the cardiac cells from the environment-controlled microscopic stage onto a television monitor (Sanyo, model VM 4155). A photodiode, which can be maneuvered to any point on the screen, detects changes in light intensity resulting from pulsations of the cells. Each beat is permanently documented through the interfacing of the photodiode to a Grass Instruments, Model 7, polygraph recorder. A schematic illustration of the system and a sample recording are shown in Figure 1.

In the polygraph recording note the consistency of beating in these noninnervated cardiac cells. To measure this consistency, a DEC PDP 11/34 computer was connected to the photodiode, which accumulated the intervals of time between beats. Figure 2 shows a histogram analysis of the intervals of time between beats, measured to within 10^{-3} seconds of cells kept at constant temperature (29±0.2°) and pH (7.4). Table 1 summarizes the results of four such measurements at temperatures ranging from 29.5 to 37.5°C.

The relatively small standard deviations of the intervals of time between beats at each temperature (2.04) illustrates the high degree of precision with which these cells function in the absence of neuronal control and under defined conditions of temperature and pH. Depending on seeding and growth conditions, cardiac cultures maintain rhythmic beating for months. We have kept several cultures beating for up to a year.

With the ability to maintain functionally active cardiac cells in culture for prolonged periods, we began to develop this system as an *in vitro* model to study the cardiopathogenesis produced in patients treated with the potent, broad-spectrum, anticancer agent adriamycin (ADM). The two general classes of cardiac effects produced by ADM in patients that have been described are early electrocardiographic changes, which are usually transient, not related to dose, and have not been predictive of further cardiac effects, and late appearing cardiomyopathy, which has led to fatal congestive heart failure and is dependent on the cumulative dose.[1-5] The latter effect has seriously restricted the effective long-term use of this antitumor drug.

Division of Cell Growth and Regulation, Sidney Farber Cancer Institute, and Department of Medicine, Cardiovascular Division, Brigham and Women's Hospital, Harvard Medical School, Boston, Massachusetts

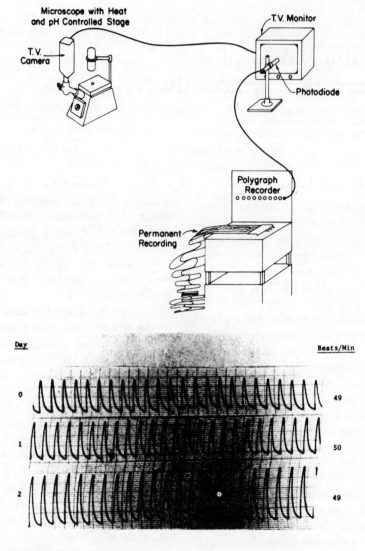

FIGURE 1. (A) Monitoring system devised to measure and record beating patterns of cardiac muscle cells in culture. (B) Sample polygraph recording.

We have recently reported that many of the structural and functional effects observed in patients and laboratory animals treated with ADM could be simulated *in vitro*.[6] Summarizing these results, we have observed that at high ADM doses (100 μg/ml) primary cardiac cell cultures derived from newborn rats ceased beating and became vacuolated within 4 hours of continuous exposure. At 24–48 hours, in drug-free medium, all cells in these cultures lysed and detached from the petri dish surfaces. At 10 μg/ml ADM for 1 hour, cardiac muscle cells undergo nucleolar fragmentation and detach from the plate surface, 48–72 hours after treatment. At 2 μg/ml of 1-hour treatment, no discernible effects of ADM could be seen for as long as the cells were maintained (10 months). At low doses (≤ 0.1 μg/ml) no immediate effects on beating or on the structure of cardiac cells could be detected by phase-

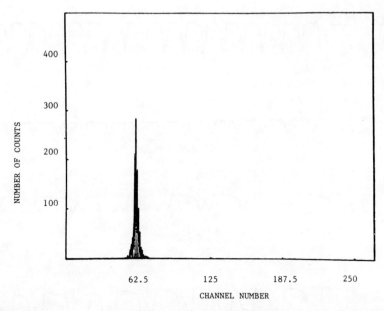

FIGURE 2. Histogram showing time intervals (within 10^{-3} sec) between beats of cardiac muscle cells in culture with constant temperature of 29 ±0.2°C and ph = 7.4.

contrast or electron microscopy. Although beating rates did in general decrease with increasing drug exposure time, the variability in the beating rates of treated cultures made this an unreliable parameter for measuring functional effects. A more consistent effect produced by continuous exposure to low doses of ADM was arrhythmia. Both the incidence and apparent severity of arrhthymias followed a dose-dependent course. Thus at 3 days of continuous treatment, 4 of 11 treated cultures showed arrhythmia at the highest dose (0.1 µg/ml), while at the lowest dose (0.05 µg/ml) only 1 of 10 cultures became arrhythmic. At 5 days of continuous treatment, all 11 cultures treated with 0.1 µg/ml were arrhythmic, while 6 of 10 treated with 0.05 µg/ml had become arrhythmic at this time. At 9 days of continuous exposure, all of the treated cultures became arrhythmic, while 10 of 10 untreated cultures continued to beat rhythmically. Figure 3 is an illustration of the difference in arrhythmic patterns at two distinct dose levels. At 0.01 µg/ml, no effects on rhythmicity could be detected, while at 0.05 µg/ml at 2 days of exposure, individual cultures beat with double contractions. Although normal single pulsations were interrupted at this dose level, the interval of time between each set of double contractions remained consistent. At twice the dose (0.1 µg/ml) the interval of time between double pulsations became irregular. These two types of irregular beating patterns were reversible at 48 hours of drug treatment, when cells were rinsed and reincubated in drug-free medium and the cells remained morphologically intact

TABLE 1. Summary of Four Measurements of Beating of Noninnervated Cardiac Cells

Number of Counts	Temperature (°C)	Average Beats/ Minute	Standard Deviation
1000	29.6	61.9	0.86
1000	33.0	99.9	2.04
1000	34.8	108.6	0.62
1000	35.9	128.2	2.04

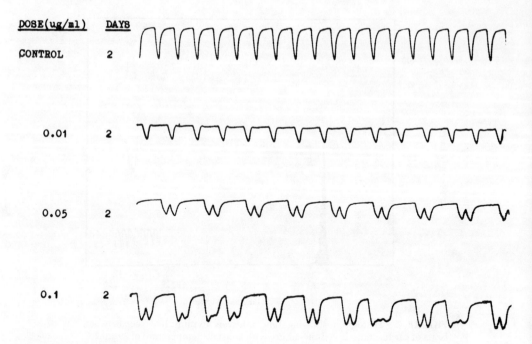

FIGURE 3.   Adriamycin continuous treatment. Polygraph recording (10 mm/sec chart speed) of cultures continuously exposed to ADM for 2 days at different dose levels. The 15-second tracings shown here are representative of the beating patterns of cultures that were each monitored for 8 minutes.

for the remainder of the experiment (2 weeks). However, when cultures were continuously exposed to 0.1 μg/ml ADM for prolonged periods (>2 weeks), severe loss of muscle fiber/muscle cell was observed by both phase-contrast and electron microscopy. It was determined that greater than 95% of the muscle cells underwent this loss. In contrast to the pathology produced at high-dose ADM, vacuolization and nucleolar fragmentation were not observed at low-dose, long-term treatment.

Thus, utilizing this *in vitro* system, we could not only produce several of the structural and functional ADM-induced cardiac effects reported *in vivo*, but could distinguish between high- and low-dose pathology as well as determine and separate doses that produce reversible-functional effects from those that produce irreversible structural damage.

Recently, several independent studies have indicated a reduction in cardiomyopathy in patients treated with fractionated doses of ADM.[7-9] Although the high doses used in our *in vitro* system, which produce vacuolization, nucleolar fragmentation, and myocytolysis, are higher than those reported *in vivo*, it is conceivable that the reduced cardiac toxicity reported with fractionated doses in the clinic may result from the absence of the high-dose pathology.

We have recently observed immediate reversal of ADM-induced arrhythmias by colchicine and vinblastine, compounds known to exert effects on microtubule assembly and on Ca^{2+} transport. Since Ca^{2+} transport has been shown to be altered by ADM treatment,[10] this latter effect of colchicine and vinblastine may be involved in the reversal of ADM-induced arrhythmia. Figure 4 is an illustration of the beat-

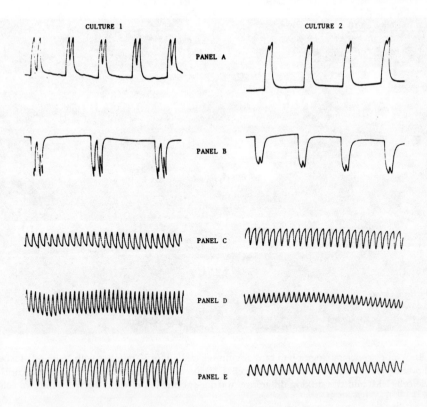

FIGURE 4.   Reversal of ADM-induced arrhythmias by vinblastine. Beating patterns of cardiac cell cultures (1 and 2) treated continuously with ADM (0.2 µg/ml) for 24 hours (Panel A) and 48 hours (Panel B). Vinblastine (16 µ g/ml) was added and the beating patterns were recorded 20 seconds (Panel C), 3 minutes (Panel D), and 24 hours (Panel E) later.

ing patterns of two individual cultures treated with ADM for 24 hours and subsequently treated with vinblastine (16 µg/ml). The reversal to single rhythmic pulsations was almost immediate and cells continued to beat rhythmically for the remainder of the experiment (24 hours). When cultures were washed free of both ADM and vinblastine (48 hours later), they continued to beat rhythmically.

Intracellular Localization and Accumulation

Cardiac cultures contain mixed populations of muscle and nonmuscle cells, which are easily distinguishable. By use of the inherent fluorescence of ADM, we have recently observed increased nuclear accumulation of ADM fluorescence and a corresponding increase in nucleolar fragmentation in cardiac muscle as compared to nonmuscle cells.[11]

In cultures treated for 30 minutes with 10 µg/ml of ADM both nonmuscle and muscle cells show a distinct drug fluorescence localized in the nucleus, with little fluorescence in the cytoplasm. A striking difference in staining was noted, however, with cardiac muscle nuclei showing a significantly greater intensity of anthracycline-specific fluorescence as compared to nonmuscle cell nuclei (Fig. 5). With prolonged exposure, ADM-associated fluorescence appeared in the cytoplasm of both cell types. The fluorescence appeared in discrete areas of the cytoplasm, which, as could be determined by phase-contrast

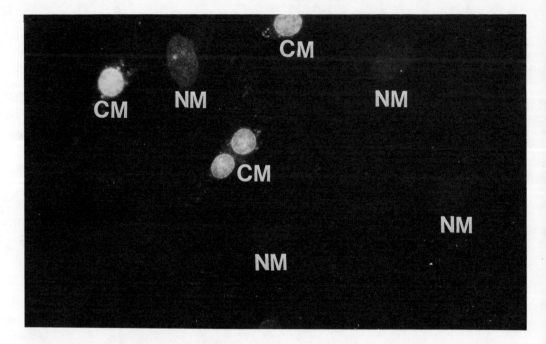

FIGURE 5. Fluorescence micrograph of cardiac cultures treated for 30 minutes with 10 μg/ml of ADM. Note the small rounded nuclei of the cardiac muscle cell (CM) as compared to the larger oval-shaped nuclei in the nonmuscle cell (NM) and the striking difference in drug-specific fluorescence between the two cell types.

microscopy, did not correspond to mito-chondrial areas.

By rinsing cells after short drug ex-posures (30 minutes) and incubating in drug-free medium, it was determined that the loss of drug from the nucleus was con-tributing to the appearance of cytoplasmic staining. After prolonged incubation peri-ods in drug-free medium (24 hours), nu-clear and cytoplasmic staining was still evident in cardiac muscle cells, whereas little if any diffuse cytoplasmic staining could be detected in nonmuscle cells. The nonmuscle cell nuclei had become free of fluorescence staining at 6 hours in drug-free medium.

Concomitant with intercellular differ-ences in drug-associated nuclear fluores-cence, a selective effect on nucleoli was observed in muscle as compared to non-muscle cells. Nucleolar fragmentation was seen in muscle cell nucleoli 24 hours fol-lowing a 30 minute exposure to ADM,

while the nucleoli of nonmuscle cells were intact.

In order to determine whether the selec-tive cardiac nuclear accumulation was a general property of anthracyclines or whether it was restricted to ADM, a number of anthracyclines already tested in animals were examined in our *in vitro* sys-tem. Figures 6–9 are matched fluorescence and phase-contrast micrographs of cells treated with 10 μg/ml for 30 minutes of detorubicin, rubidazone, daunorubicin, and N-leucyldaunorubicin, respectively, all kindly provided by Dr. Rene Maral of L'Institut de Cancérologie et d'immuno-génétique, Villejuif, France. In each of the first three fluorescence micrographs it can be seen that these compounds are localized mainly in the nucleus and also fluoresce more in cardiac muscle than nonmuscle cell nuclei. Interestingly, N-leucyldauno-rubicin (Fig. 9), which appears less toxic than the other compounds in our *in vitro*

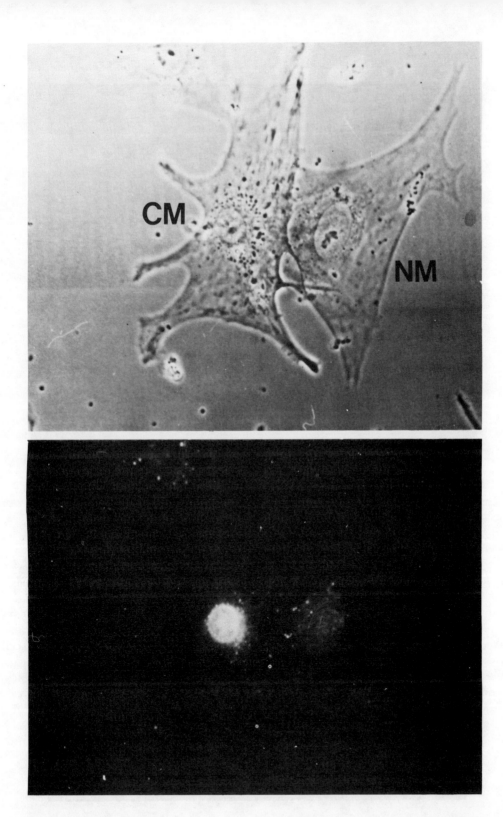

FIGURE 6. Matched phase-contrast and fluorescence micrographs of cardiac cultures treated for 30 minutes with 10 μg/ml of detorubicin. Note the difference in drug-specific fluorescence between the two cell types.

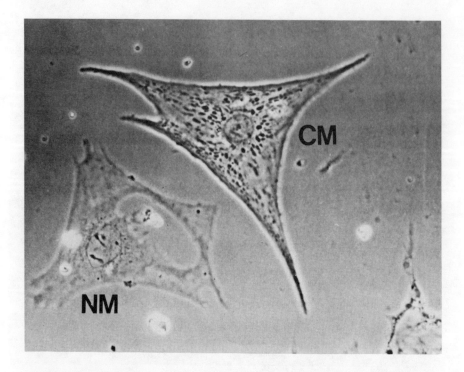

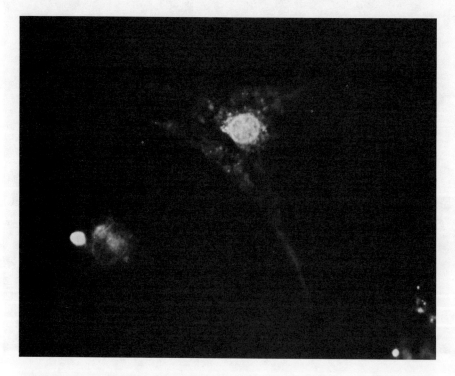

FIGURE 7. Matched phase-contrast and fluorescence micrographs of cardiac cultures treated for 30 minutes with 10 μg/ml of rubidazone. Note the difference in drug-specific fluorescence between the two cell types.

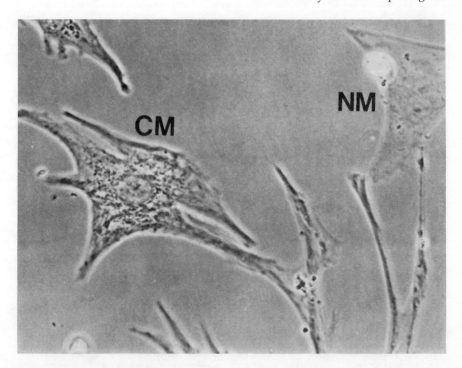

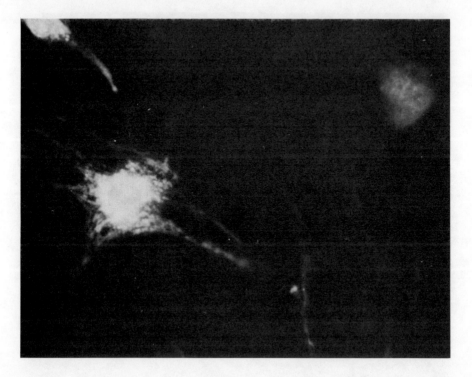

FIGURE 8. Matched phase-contrast and fluorescence micrographs of cardiac cultures treated for 30 minutes with 10 μg/ml of daunorubicin. Note the difference in drug-specific fluorescence between the two cell types and also the appearance of cytoplasmic as well as nuclear staining.

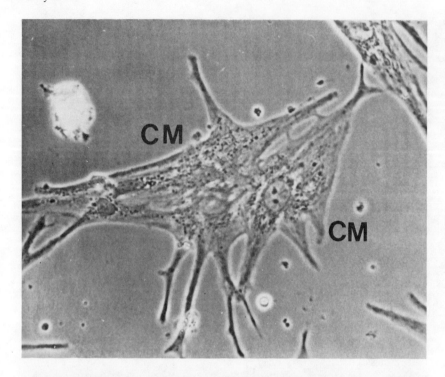

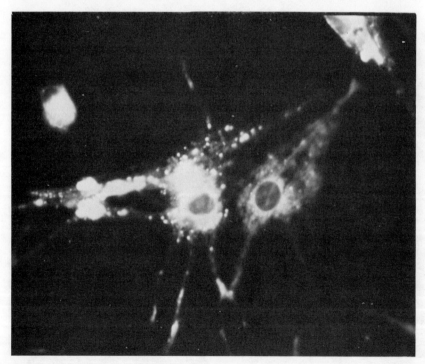

FIGURE 9.   Matched phase-contrast and fluorescence micrographs of cardiac cultures treated for 30 minutes with 10 μg/ml of N-leucyldaunorubicin. Note the absence of nuclear staining in the cardiac muscle cells.

system, localizes in the cytoplasm (and does not stain nuclei) in both cardiac muscle and nonmuscle cells. The two other anthracycline analogues we have examined, which have been reported to have less cardiotoxicity than ADM *in vivo*, N-trifluoroacetyladriamycin-14-valerate (AD-32) and its polar analogue, AD-143, also localize in the cytoplasm. In addition, we could not detect preferential accumulation in cardiac muscle cells with these three cytoplasmic-localizing analogues.

Thus we have identified three more anthracyclines that show preferential nuclear accumulation in cardiac muscle cell nuclei. These three compounds also display similar toxicities relative to those determined for ADM, i.e., a 10-μg/ml 1-hour treatment kills cardiac muscle cells 48–72 hours later. It must be emphasized, however, that these results are preliminary, and, until we test a substantial number of compounds for localization, preferential uptake, and subsequent toxicity, the *in vivo* significance of our *in vitro* observations remain uncertain.

In summary, we have demonstrated that cardiac muscle cells *in vitro*, in the absence of neuronal control, display remarkable precision in their ability to beat autorhythmically. Utilizing these cells, we have established that many of the structural and functional cardiac effects induced in patients receiving ADM chemotherapy and in treated laboratory animals can be simulated *in vitro*. The structural effects of vacuolization and nucleolar fragmentation were seen only at high doses, at relatively short incubation times (48 hours), whereas significant loss of muscle fiber/muscle cell was observed at low doses after prolonged treatment in culture (17 days). Thus, the two structural effects, vacuolization and loss of muscle fiber, reported to be an accurate means of assessing cardiac damage in patients receiving ADM treatment,[12] could be shown to occur at distinct dose levels in culture. This finding may have relevance to the reported decrease in car-

diotoxicity of patients receiving intermittent low doses of ADM compared to those receiving the standard bolus injections. In the former case the high-dose pathological effects of ADM may have been eliminated.

Additionally, we have demonstrated that colchicine and vinblastine, two compounds that effect Ca^{2+} transport in cells, can reverse the low-dose arrhythmias produced *in vitro*. We plan a series of experiments to determine whether these compounds will reduce the effects of ADM and its related analogues on the structural integrity of the cardiac muscle cell. Also, through the use of our electronic monitoring system, we plan to determine by use of known antiarrhythmic agents the precise nature of each of the identified patterns of arrhythmia.

Consistent with our observation of preferential ADM-accumulation by muscle cell nuclei in cardiac cells in culture, an increase in ADM-induced nuclear fragmentation in muscle cells was observed relative to nonmuscle cells. This finding may have relevance with respect to ADM-induced cardiotoxicity *in vivo*. The preliminary data presented concerning several known cardiotoxic and noncardiotoxic anthracyclines suggests a correlation between *in vitro* cardiac cell toxicity and *in vivo* cardiotoxicity. The observed increase in nuclear accumulation of ADM in cardiac muscle cells has now been demonstrated for several other cardiotoxic anthracyclines. The possibility exists that preferential accumulation may contribute to *in vivo* cardiopathogenesis, even though to date there has been no demonstration of preferential cardiac accumulation of ADM *in vivo*. One possible explanation for this discrepancy may involve the differences in nuclear distribution among various tissues. Since cardiac muscle cells in culture contain smaller nuclei than the other cell types studied, the differences in total tissue uptake *in vivo* may be dependent upon the amount of nuclear material in the different tissues used for comparison.

Obviously, in the selection of new anthracycline fermentation products and synthetic analogues for preclinical development and initial clinical trial, the evaluation of potential cardiac toxicity or lack thereof is an important determinant. Each of the experimental animal models used to date (rabbit, monkey, hamster, rat, and mouse) exhibits one or more serious drawbacks relating either to cost or scientific value. The cardiac cell culture system, which requires only milligram quantities of test agent, offers the advantages of studying direct effects of these agents at the cellular and subcellular level. In addition, it is a simpler, more rapid, and far less expensive means than any *in vivo* model for evaluating the potential effects of anthracycline agents on the heart.

ACKNOWLEDGMENTS

This work was supprted by a Young Investigator Award from the National Cancer Institute, CA 24771.

REFERENCES

1. Gilladoga AC, Manuel C, Tan C, Wollner N, Murphy LM: Cardiotoxicity of adriamycin in children. *Cancer Chemother Rep 6: 209–214, 1975.*
2. Minow RA, Benjamin RS, Gottlieb JA: Adriamycin cardiomyopathy: An overview with determination of risk factors. *Cancer Chemother Rep 6: 195–201, 1975.*
3. Bonadonna G, Beretta G, Tancici G, Brambilla C, Bajetta E, DePalo GM, Del Lena M, Fossati Bellani F, Gasparini M, Valagussa P, Veronesi U: Adriamycin studies at the Istituto Nazionale Tumori, Milan. *Cancer Chemother Rep 6: 231–245, 1975.*
4. Cortes EP, Lutman G, Wanka J, Wang JJ, Pickren J, Wallace J, Holland JF: Adriamycin cardiotoxicity: A clinicopathologic correlation. *Cancer Chemother Rep 6: 215–225, 1975.*
5. Lefrak EA, Pitha J, Rosenheim S, Gottleib JA: A clinicopathologic correlation. *Cancer 32: 302–314, 1973.*
6. Lampidis TJ, Henderson IC, Israel M, Canellos GP: Structural and functional effects of adriamycin on cardiac cells *in vitro. Cancer Res 40: 3901–3909, 1980.*
7. Weiss AJ, Manthei RW: Experience with the use of adriamycin in combination with other anticancer agents using a weekly schedule, with particular reference to lack of cardiac toxicity. *Cancer 40: 2046–2052, 1977.*
8. Lazarus AJ, Manthei RW: Experience with the use of adriamycin in combination with other anticancer agents using a weekly schedule, with particular reference to lack of cardiac toxicity. *Cancer 40: 2046–2052, 1977.*
9. Von Hoff DD, Layand M, Basa P, Davis HL Jr., Von Hoff AL, Rozenweig M, Muggia FM: Risk factors for doxorubicin-induced congestive heart failure. *Ann Intern Med 91: 710–717, 1979.*
10. Villani R, Piccinini F, Merelli P, Faualli L: Influence of adriamycin on calcium exchangeability in cardiac muscle and its modification by ouabain. *Biochem Pharmacol 27: 985–987, 1978.*
11. Lampidis TJ, Johnson LV, Israel M: Effects of adriamycin on rat heart cells in culture: Increased accumulation and nucleoli fragmentation in cardiac muscle vs non-muscle cells. *J Mol Cell Cardiol 13: 913–924, 1981.*
12. Billingham M, Bristow ME, Mason JW, Daniels JR: Anthracycline cardiomyopathy monitored by morphologic changes. *Cancer Treat Rep 62: 857–864, 1978.*

CHAPTER 7

Cardiotoxicity Models

G. Zbinden

Animal models for drug-induced human diseases must serve many purposes: they may be used in an effort to establish the causal role of the chemical, to elucidate the biological mechanisms, to provide information on structure–activity relationships for the chemist working in synthetic drugs, to identify chemicals that enhance or antagonize the undesirable characteristics of a drug, and to investigate the importance of metabolic and pharmacokinetic factors. Depending on the interests of the investigators, experimental models are developed that are particularly suited to answer specific questions.

In the case of anthracycline cardiotoxicity, it was first necessary to confirm the clinical observations of cardiotoxic properties and to establish the causal role of the drugs. For this purpose, whole animal models were looked for with which the development of the myocardial lesion could be followed. It was found that the rabbit and the monkey were particularly well suited, since the cardiac damage was readily induced and closely resembled that observed in man.[11,15] For biomechanistic investigations, in vitro models are often more useful. With cardiotoxic anthracyclines, a variety of biological effects were discovered, such as depression of ADP-stimulated mitochondrial respiration,[1,2] uncoupling of oxidative phosphorylation,[2] and enhanced Ca^{2+} influx through slow channels into the cells of perfused chicken hearts.[1] These studies were, in part, extended to ex vivo experiments that showed that the electron transport mechanisms and coupling of oxidative phosphorylation in mitochondria isolated from hearts of anthracycline-treated rats were impaired and that Ca^{2+} uptake into mitochondria was enhanced.[2,3]

Pharmacokinetic and metabolic studies also contributed to the understanding of anthracycline cardiotoxicity. For example, N,N-dimethyldoxorubicin (NSC-261045), which differed from doxorubicin only by a dimethyl substitution at the daunosamine moiety, exhibited greatly enhanced cardiotoxicity in rats, an effect that could be explained by a much higher accumulation of this compound in the heart.[21] On the other hand, N-L-leucyldaunorubicin accumulated less in the heart of rabbits and was clearly less cardiotoxic in the rabbit model than doxorubicin and daunorubicin.[10]

Toxicological Screening for New Anthracyclines

Thanks to their potent and broad-spectrum antitumor activity, the anthracyclines have gained an important place in cancer chemotherapy. Unfortunately, cardiotoxic properties prevent their unconditioned use, and therapy must always be discontinued at a certain point to prevent the development of fatal cardiomyopathy. Therefore the development of less cardiotoxic analogues is of utmost importance. Since synthetic and semisynthetic anthracyclines are difficult to make and costly, it is essential to have animal models that can recognize and quantify cardiotoxic proper-

Institute of Toxicology, Swiss Federal Institute of Technology and University of Zurich, Schwerzenbach, Switzerland

49

ties of new substances rapidly, and with small expense for the newly synthesized test drugs.

In recent years, the rat has become more and more accepted as a useful animal species for the toxicological assessment of new anthracyclines. Repeated administration of such drugs produces characteristic ultrastructural lesions of the myocardium of the rat, even at doses that do not severely impair general health and do not fatally depress bone marrow function.[13,14,20] However, it requires careful and prolonged dosing to induce such morphological lesions. Moreover, since the myocardial damage is focal, it is quite difficult and time consuming to assess it quantitatively by morphometric evaluation of the ultrastructural changes. In an effort to find a more readily measurable cardiotoxic effect of anthracyclines the usefulness of serial electrocardiography was explored. It was found that repeated I.P. injections of doxorubicin and related drugs in rats caused significant and characteristic changes of the electrocardiogram (ECG) already in the early stages of treatment. The most conspicuous effect was progressive widening of the QRS complex, a change that was highly reproducible and that could, thus, be used as a screening parameter for the cardiotoxic effect of new anthracyclines.[20,23]

In order to quantify the cardiotoxic characteristics of anthracyclines in the rat screening model the minimal cumulative cardiotoxic dose (MCCD), defined as the cumulative dose per kilogram of body weight causing significant widening of the QRS complex, was introduced. In many experiments with doxorubicin the MCCD was found to vary between 8 and 12 mg/kg. Rubidazone and N-L-leucyldaunorubicin (RP 20 132) had a MCCD of approximately 24 mg/kg.[18,20] With the latter compound, it was found that the ECG changes were mild, even at a cumulative dose of 40 mg/kg. It was, thus, concluded that rubidazone and particularly the N-L-leucyl analogue were significantly less car-

diotoxic than doxorubicin on a weight for weight basis. For RP 20 132, this conclusion was recently confirmed in chronic rabbit experiments,[10] and for rubidazone a considerably higher cardiotoxic dose than that of doxorubicin was determined in human subjects, using appearance of ultrastructural lesions in endomyocardial biopsies as an indicator.[4]

Up to now, 70 new anthracyclines have been evaluated in the rat screening model for cardiotoxicity. The most rapid results were obtained with highly cardiotoxic compounds, such as the N,N-dimethyldoxorubicin, referred to above.[21] With such agents, characteristic ECG changes occurred usually within 1 week. With less cardiotoxic compounds, treatment had to be continued for up to 3 weeks and doses were increased gradually. But in most cases it has been possible to arrive at a preliminary assessment of the cardiotoxic properties of a new derivative using less than 100 mg.[20]

In order to illustrate the usefulness of this screening method the results with several rubidazone derivatives modified in the benzhydrazone side chain may be mentioned. With these drugs, a statistically significant correlation between the cardiotoxic properties in the rat model and the electronic characteristics of the side chain could be demonstrated.[16] Since these derivatives were all highly active as antitumor agents, the chemical modification resulted in a definite improvement of the therapeutic index.

The study of many anthracyclines has clearly shown that chemotherapeutic activities in various animal tumor models and cardiotoxicity in the rat screening system are not highly correlated. For example, appreciable cardiotoxicity was demonstrated with compounds that were inactive as antitumor drugs in the P388 mouse leukemia model. Other compounds that were at least as active as doxorubicin as antitumor agents were up to 10-fold less cardiotoxic in the rat.[20] From these observations, it is concluded that it should be possible to separate antitumor activity and cardiotoxic properties, at least to a considerable degree.

Evaluation of New Types of Anthracyclines and Anthracyclinelike Drugs

The search for new anthracyclines is not limited to derivatives of the standard agents daunorubicin and doxorubicin, but has been extended to antibiotics produced by other microorganisms. An example is carminomycin, a compound isolated from cultures of *Actinomadura carminata*. Preliminary clinical studies have indicated low potential for cardiotoxicity.[6]

In the rat screening model, carminomycin did not induce the characteristic widening of the QRS complex, at least as long as the animals were in good general condition. Electron microscopy of the myocardial tissue disclosed mostly loss of myofibrillar mass but no dilatation of the sarcotubular system which is characteristic of anthracycline cariomyopathy. Therefore it was concluded that carminomycin caused mostly a cardiac atrophy, probably as a consequence of inhibition of protein synthesis. This effect on the heart is less specific than that observed with doxorubicin and related compounds. It is likely that the compound will not be as damaging to the human heart as the anthracyclines derived from *Streptomyces peucetius* var. *caesius*.[19]

Another compound derived from a different microorganism is cinerubin A. This drug induced rapid and marked ECG changes in rats, including in some instances marked elevation of the ST segment and extreme distortion of the QRS complex. These animals showed marked, infarct-like lesions of the myocardium. Thus this compound proved to be highly cardiotoxic in the rat model system, and its further development was discouraged.[17]

In recent years several groups have attempted to synthesize anthracycline-like drugs. Of these, a series of anthracenediones have received some attention. The compounds are highly active in the antitumor screening models, and they often exhibit cross-resistance in anthracycline-resistant P388 mouse leukemia sublines.[5]

Preliminary studies of two of these anthracenediones (NSC-196473 and NSC-287513) have shown that the compounds did not induce the characteristic ECG changes seen with cardiotoxic anthracyclines, at least as long as well-tolerated doses were given. Electron microscopic evaluation of the heart did not disclose the typical lesion seen with cardiotoxic anthracyclines, but the compounds appeared to affect mostly mitochondrial structure.[5,18] From these preliminary findings, it appears that the anthracenediones studied so far differed from doxorubicin and related compounds with regard to their cardiotoxic properties. As was found with carminomycin, the anthracenediones seem to be less specifically cardiotoxic than anthracyclines; therefore their clinical evaluation is of greatest interest.

Discovery of Anthracycline Antagonists

An attractive possibility to reduce the hazard of anthracycline therapy would be the use of drugs that counteract the cardiotoxic effect without interfering with the chemotherapeutic activity. The rat cardiotoxicity model is well suited to study such compounds. For example, coenzyme Q10 given in equimolar doses with doxorubicin inhibited the development of ECG changes.[22] This compound was also shown to counteract the inhibition of cardiac succineoxidase and of NADH oxidase by cardiotoxic anthracyclines *in vitro*.[12] Its potential for counteracting anthracycline heart damage in man is at present under investigation.

A marked antagonistic effect against doxorubicin-induced cardiomyopathy in rats was observed with the antitumor drug ICRF-159. This compound was selected because it prevented an increase of coronary perfusion pressure in the isolated dog heart caused by daunorubicin and doxorubicin[9] and because it reduced drastically acute daunorubicin toxicity in various laboratory animal species.[8,17] In the repeated dose experiment in rats, it was found that the drug increased the depressant effect of doxorubicin on bone marrow and lymphatic tissue. It is, thus, likely that the antitumor effects of the two agents are additive. On the other hand, the cardiotoxic effects of doxorubicin were antagonized.[19] The mechanism of action of this antagonism is not explained. However, it should be noted that ICRF-159 is a chelator of Ca^{2+} ions. Since, as it was pointed out above, anthracycline antibiotics enhance the influx of Ca^{2+} ions through slow channels,[1] and since calcium overload is likely to disturb metabolic processes in the myocytes[1] it is understandable that chelation of Ca^{2+} ions may counteract these processes and may thus prevent the development of myocardial damage. The experiment demonstrating the antagonistic effect of ICRF-159 in rats is presently repeated.

If the results of the first study can be confirmed, it would be desirable to explore the ICRF-159 and doxorubicin combination also in man.

Conclusion

The development of animal models for the evaluation of the cardiotoxic effects of anthracycline antibiotics has been of great importance for the understanding of the undesirable effects of this valuable class of therapeutic agents. For the development of new derivatives and new types of anthracycline-like drugs and for the discovery of potential anthracycline antagonists, these animal models have become valuable tools without which the directed chemical synthesis would be impossible. It is hoped that the toxicological models in which structural, functional, and biochemical lesions induced by anthracyclines can be assessed will lead to the discovery of new compounds with high chemotherapeutic activity and greatly reduced potential for myocardial damage.

ACKNOWLEDGMENTS

Research reported in this paper was supported by a grant from the Swiss National Science Foundation. Many of the drugs studied were provided by the Drug Synthesis and Chemistry Branch, Developmental Therapeutics Program, Division of Cancer Treatment, National Cancer Institute, Silver Spring, Maryland, under contract number 236-77-C-0410 CC.

REFERENCES

1. Azuma J, Sperelakis N, Hasegawa H, Tanimoto T, Vogel S, Ogura K, Awata N, Sawamura A, Harada H, Ishiyamo T, Morita Y, Yamamora Y: Adriamycin cardiotoxicity: Possible pathogenetic mechanisms. *J Mol Cell Cardiol* 13: 381–397, 1981.
2. Bachmann E, Weber E, Zbinden G: Effects of seven anthracycline antibiotics on electrocardiogram and mitochondrial function of rat hearts. *Agents Actions* 4: 383–393, 1974.
3. Bachmann E, Zbinden G: Effect of doxorubicin and rubidazone on respiratory function and Ca^{2+} transport in rat heart mitochondria. *Toxicol Lett* 3: 29–34, 1979.
4. Benjamin RS, Mason JW, Billingham ME: Cardiac toxicity of adriamycin-DNA complex and rubidazone: Evaluation by electrocardiogram and endomyocardial biopsy. *Cancer Treat Rep* 62: 935–939, 1978.
5. Cheng CC, Ing RB, Wood HB Jr, Zbinden G, Zee-Cheng RKY: Comparison of antineoplastic activity of aminoethylaminoanthraquinones and the anthracycline antibiotics. *J Pharmacol Sci* 68: 393–396, 1979.
6. Crooke ST: A review of carminomycin — a new anthracycline developed in the USSR. *J Med* 8: 295–316, 1977.
7. Fleckenstein A, Janke J, Dörig HJ, Leder O: Key role of Ca in the production of noncoronarogenic myocardial necrosis. In *Recent Advances in Studies of Cardiac Structure and Metabolism. Vol. 6. Pathophysiology and Morphology of Myocardial Cell Alterations.* Fleckenstein A, Rona G, (Eds), University Park Press, Baltimore, 1974, pp 21–32.
8. Herman EH, Mhatre RM, Chadwick DP: Modification of some of the toxic effects of daunomycin (NSC-82151) by treatment with the antineoplastic agent ICRF 159 (NSC-129943). *Toxicol Appl Pharmacol* 27: 517–526, 1974.
9. Hermann EH, Mhatre RM, Lee IP, Waravdekar

US: Prevention of the cardiotoxic effects of adriamycin and daunomycin in the isolated dog heart. *Proc Soc Exp Biol Med 140: 234–239, 1972*.

10. Jaenke RS, Deprez-De Campeneere D, Truet A: Cardiotoxicity and comparative pharmacokinetics of six anthracyclines in the rabbit. *Cancer Res 40: 3530–3536, 1980*.

11. Jaenke RS: An anthracycline antibiotic-induced cardiomyopathy in rabbits. *Lab Invest 30: 292–304, 1974*.

12. Kishi T, Kishi H, Folkers K: Inhibition of cardiac Co Q10-enzymes by clinically used drugs and possible prevention. In *Biomedical and Clinical Aspects of Coenzyme Q*. Folkers K, Yamamora Y, (Eds), Elsevier North-Holland Biomedical Press, Amsterdam, 1977, pp 47—62.

13. Mettler FP, Young DM, Ward JM: Adriamycin-induced cardiotoxicity (cardiomyopathy and congestive heart failure) in rats. *Cancer Res 37: 2705–2713, 1977*.

14. Olson HM: The rat as a model system in evaluating anthracycline cardiotoxicity. In *Anthracyclines: Current Status and New Developments. Crooke ST, Reich SD, (Eds), Academic Press, New York, 1980, pp 171–191*.

15. Schmidt LH: The cardiotoxicity of adriamycin as exhibited in the rhesus monkey. Paper presented at the Working Symposium on Anthracycline Antibiotics, National Cancer Institute, Division of Cancer Treatment April 22–23, 1976.

16. Tong GL, Cory M, Lee WW, Henry DW, Zbinden G: Antitumor anthracycline antibiotics. Structure–activity and structure–cardiotoxicity relationships of rubidazone analogues. *J Med Chem 21: 732–737, 1978*.

17. Woodman RJ, Cysyk RL, Kline I, Gang M, Venditti JM: Enhancement of the effectiveness of daunorubicin (NSC-82151) or adriamycin (NSC-129943) against early mouse L1210 leukemia with ICRF-159 (NSC-129943). *Cancer Chemother Rep 59: 689–696, 1975*.

18. Zbinden G: Unpublished results, 1981.

19. Zbinden G: Assessment of cardiotoxic effects in chronic rat toxicity studies. In *Cardiac Toxicity*. Balazs T, (Ed), CRC Press, Boca Raton, Fla, 1980.

20. Zbinden G, Bachmann E, Holderegger C: Model systems for cardiotoxic effects of anthracyclines. *Antibiot Chemother 23: 255–270, 1978*.

21. Zbinden G, Pfister M, Holderegger C: Cardiotoxicity of N,N-dimethyladriamycin (NSC-261045) in rats. *Toxicol Lett 1: 267–274, 1978*.

22. Zbinden G, Bachmann E, Bolliger H: Study of coenzyme Q in toxicity of adriamycin. In *Biomedical and Clinical Aspects of Coenzyme Q*. Folkers K, Yamamura Y, (Eds), Elsevier/North Holland Biomedical Press, Amsterdam, 1977, pp 219–228.

23. Zbinden G, Brändle E: Toxicologic screening of daunorubicin (NSC-82151), adriamycin (NSC-123127), and their derivatives in rats. *Cancer Chemother Rep 59: 707–715, 1975*.

CHAPTER 8

Mechanisms of Anthracycline-Mediated Cardiotoxicity

R. A. Newman and M. P. Hacker

Despite a sizable recent increase in the literature concerned with proposed mechanisms of cardiotoxicity produced by anthracyclines, no single hypothesis has yet been universally accepted that adequately explains the unique cardiac toxicity of this class of oncolytic drugs. As Myers[1] has pointed out in a recent review, much of the literature on anthracycline-mediated toxicity tends to be phenomenological in nature. It is therefore difficult at present to conclude whether one or several of the pharmacological effects produced by anthracyclines are involved separately in the drug-mediated antitumor and cardiotoxic responses or whether the same mechanisms that are involved in the antitumor response also mediate the cardiomyopathic effects.

Anthracycline cardiomyopathy is now known to represent two types of reactions characterized by early, transient electrocardiographic alterations or acute changes and a delayed progressive cardiomyopathy that have been well defined with regard to histopathological changes in human beings as well as several laboratory animals and *in vitro* culture model systems. It is the chronic cardiomyopathy that remains as one of the most negative attributes of the anthracycline class of oncolytic drugs. Most of the research aimed at defining the mechanisms of anthracycline

cardiotoxicity has therefore been conducted in attempts at explaining the chronic rather than the acute drug-mediated cardiomyopathic changes. An outline of proposed cellular sites that are believed to be important in the development of the chronic phase of anthracycline-mediated cardiotoxicity is presented in Figure 1.

Chronic Indirect Effects

A possible indirect drug-mediated mechanism for the chronic development of cardiotoxicity involves the release of vasoactive amines by such drugs as adriamycin. Bristow *et al.*[2,3] have shown that anthracyclines can cause the release of both histamine and epinephrine and have proposed that it is the combined action of these agents and possibly certain prostaglandins that is responsible for histopathologic changes typically seen with the chronic administration of adriamycin. As Myers[1] has recently pointed out, however, there are a number of problems with this proposed mechanism of anthracycline cardiotoxicity. Exposure of both myocardial cell and organ cultures to adriamycin, for example, results in the same typical histopathological changes as those observed in hearts from chronically treated animal models. Because vasocative amines are absent from these *in vitro* cardiac systems, drug-mediated damage observed *in vivo* cannot be solely ascribed to the effects of the release of histamine and epinephrine.

Vermont Regional Cancer Center, Department of Pharmacology, College of Medicine, University of Vermont, Burlington, Vermont

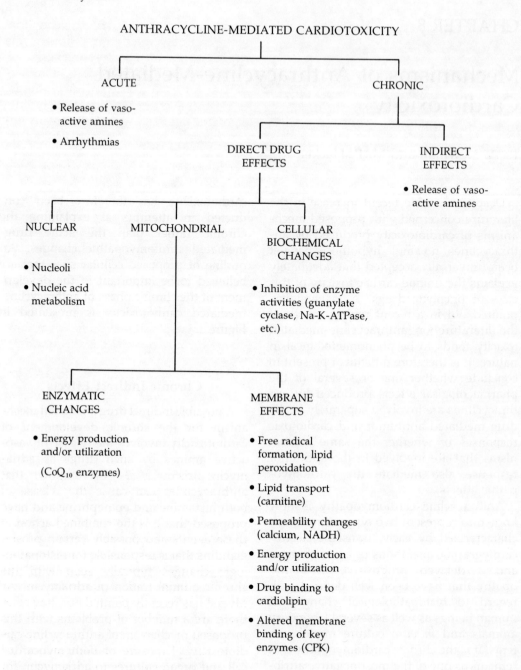

ANTHRACYCLINE-MEDIATED CARDIOTOXICITY

ACUTE

- Release of vaso-
active amines

- Arrhythmias

CHRONIC

DIRECT DRUG
EFFECTS

INDIRECT
EFFECTS

- Release of vaso-
active amines

NUCLEAR

- Nucleoli

- Nucleic acid
metabolism

MITOCHONDRIAL

CELLULAR
BIOCHEMICAL
CHANGES

- Inhibition of enzyme
activities (guanylate
cyclase, Na-K-ATPase,
etc.)

ENZYMATIC
CHANGES

- Energy production
and/or utilization

$(CoQ_{10}$ enzymes)

MEMBRANE
EFFECTS

- Free radical
formation, lipid
peroxidation

- Lipid transport
(carnitine)

- Permeability changes
(calcium, NADH)

- Energy production
and/or utilization

- Drug binding to
cardiolipin

- Altered membrane
binding of key
enzymes (CPK)

FIGURE 1. An outline of proposed cellular targets for drug interaction which are believed to be important in the development of anthracycline-mediated cardiotoxicity.

In contrast to indirect mechanisms of drug toxicity, knowledge of direct anthracycline-mediated changes in myocardial tissue is much more extensive. As seen in Figure 1, these can be most simply categorized as drug-mediated nuclear, mitochondrial, and specific cellular biochemical changes, all of which have been implicated to some extent as important causes of anthracycline cardiotoxicity.

Chronic Direct Effects

NUCLEAR CHANGES

Early work on the pathogenesis of anthracycline cardiomyopathy focused on nuclear morphological and biochemical alterations. Rosenhoff et al.,[4] for example, reported that ^{3}H-thymidine incorporation into the cardiac muscle of mice was inhibited in a dose-dependent manner by adriamycin and that this inhibition paralleled the expression of fatal toxicity. These authors implied that fatal toxicity was related to cardiac injury and that the effects on DNA synthesis were in some way related to cardiotoxicity. It is not clear, however, what kind of DNA synthesis (e.g., mitochondrial, unscheduled repair) or what specific tissue type (e.g., vascular versus muscular) actually contributed to the observed changes in DNA metabolism.[5,6]

Using singly isolated myocardial cells in culture, Lampidis et al.[7] have observed that adriamycin produces nuclear effects consisting of nucleolar segregation, fragmentation, and chromatin clumping prior to observable drug-mediated changes in mitochondrial structure. These authors point out that both nuclear and mitochondrial drug-mediated effects at early times seemed to be independent of each other. The importance of the anthracycline-mediated changes in nucleolar structure with regard to cardiac cell toxicity must, however, be questioned, since Lampidis et al. have reported that these cells were still beating even after severe nuclear changes had occurred.

In human beings, early anthracycline-mediated cardiotoxicity is characterized by myofibril loss.[8,9] Even with total myofibrillar loss, the mitochondria may retain their characteristic morphology, thereby indirectly implying that a nuclear-mediated alteration in protein synthesis may occur prior to mitochondrial effects. In addition, drug-mediated impairment of nuclear and nucleolar control of protein synthesis may result in mitochondrial damage through interference with enzyme synthesis and membrane biogenesis. As pointed out by Bristow,[3] effects of anthracyclines on myocardial protein synthesis, however, have received surprisingly little attention, despite the fact that many investigators have now shown that adriamycin and daunomycin inhibit transcription and decrease protein synthesis in heart tissue. More recently, DuVernay et al.[10] have examined the effects of anthracycline analogues with regard to whole cellular nucleic acid synthesis, nucleolar preribosomal RNA synthesis, and in vitro cytotoxicity and DNA binding abilities. Although these studies provide some insight into the mechanism of action of anthracyclines, the precise role of these drug-mediated nuclear changes in anthracycline cardiomyopathy remains unclear.

CELLULAR BIOCHEMICAL CHANGES

Drug-mediated enzymatic alterations in cardiac tissue have been implicated as having possible roles in the etiology of anthracycline cardiomyopathy. For example, Levy and coworkers[11] demonstrated a selective inhibition of rat and human cardiac guanylate (but not adenylate) cyclase activity by adriamycin. As the authors themselves point out, although cyclic guanosine monophosphate has been implicated in many biological reactions, its precise role in cell biology in general and in cardiac metabolism in particular has not yet been defined. Although some specificity of interaction with cardiac guanylate cyclase was demonstrated for anthracyclines, drug concentrations required to achieve 50% enzyme inhibition in vitro were clearly beyond those that would be achieved in vivo.

Gosalvez et al.[12] have reported that adriamycin is a potent inhibitor of both sodium-potassium-activated adenosine triphosphatase (Na-K-ATPase) of native heart microsomes and selected ion transport. They suggest that these effects may provide a basis for explaining the adriamycin cardiomyopathy as a digitalis type of toxicity. More recently, however, Solomonson and Halabrin[13] have demonstrated that adriamycin has no effect upon either ouabain-sensitive Na-K-ATPase or ouabain-insensitive ATPase activity in homogenates and microsomal fractions of cardiac tissue. These authors conclude that Na-K-ATPase is not a likely site for adriamycin-induced cardiotoxicity and present convincing arguments opposed to the findings of Gosalvez et al.[12]

Another example of a specific anthracycline-mediated alteration of cardiac enzyme function that cannot readily be categorized with regard to importance in nuclear or mitochondrial metabolism is the effect of adriamycin on cardiac metmyoglobin reductase activity. Taylor and Hochstein[14] have shown that adriamycin inhibits metmyoglobin reductase and have suggested that this inhibition may lead to a decrease in cardiac myoglobin and thus to effective cardiac hypoxia. As Myers[1] has commented, although this observation is interesting, it is not immediately apparent how this would lead to the peculiar cardiomyopathy that characterizes adriamycin.

MITOCHONDRIAL

The most commonly cited organelle believed to be involved with anthracycline-mediated cardiotoxicity is the mitochondrion. In general, studies of the effects of adriamycin and related compounds on mitochondrial structure and function can be categorized into those pertaining to drug-mediated enzymatic changes and those resulting from direct and indirect membrane effects (Fig. 1). With regard to the former category, anthracycline-mediated alteration of mitochondrial enzyme activity has been shown to result in inhibition of both energy production and utilization. One of the most significant changes observed with mitochondria from adriamycin-treated rabbits is the impairment of respiratory control, indicating damage at

the level of the electron transport chain. This may occur directly, for example, by inhibition of ubiquinone enzymes, which has been demonstrated in vitro by Ferrero et al.[15] These same authors also reported a "loosening" of the coupling of mitochondrial oxidations and an increase in mitochondrial permeability to NADH.

Yasumi et al.[16] have recently demonstrated an inhibitory action of adriamycin against two NADP-linked dehydrogenases in rat heart. Adriamycin was shown to inhibit the activity of both mitochondrial and cytoplasmic isocitrate dehydrogenases (ICDH) dose-dependently in a noncompetitive manner. Adriamycin inhibition of ICDH may have some relationship to the development of anthracycline cardiotoxicity, since this type of myocardial damage is at least partially prevented by treatment with vitamin E.[17] The authors suggest this may be important, since vitamin E deficiency induces a decrease in cardiac NADPH concentration[18] and a decrease in NADP-linked ICDH levels in cardiac tissue[19] similar to that observed in adriamycin-treated animals. Given the necessity of heart muscle to carry out oxidative phosphorylation on a continual basis, any interference with the efficiency of this process by any one or combination of enzymes involved with energy production may contribute to the specific toxic effects of anthracyclines on heart muscle.

The interaction of anthracyclines with cardiac membranes and the implications of those interactions have recently been reviewed by Myers.[1] An explanation for the affinity of anthracycline-binding to cardiac mitochondrial membranes has been offered by Duarte-Karim et al.[20] These authors have shown that adriamycin has a particularly high-binding affinity to cardiolipin, a major component of the inner mitochondrial membrane. It is not clear at present, however, whether this particular drug interaction is responsible for producing the morphologic alterations characterized in part by folded inner membranes observed in mitochondria from adria-mycin-treated animals.[21] In indirect support of this possibility, Tritton et al.[22] have recently shown a profound effect of cardiolipin on gel to liquid crystal transition temperature of liposomal membranes. The precise relationship of drug-mediated changes in mitochondrial morphology to changes in mitochondrial function, and hence to cardiac toxicity, remains to be adequately explored.

The effect of adriamycin on transmembrane ion fluxes in mitochondria has principally involved studies of calcium permeability. Several authors[23-25] have reported increased tissue calcium levels in rat and rabbit myocardium after adriamycin administration and have speculated that this might be a primary event in anthracycline cardiotoxicity. A direct inhibitory effect of adriamycin on mitochondrial calcium uptake in vitro has been shown by Moore et al.[26] However, the relation between this in vitro biochemical phenomenon and the development of drug-induced cardiomyopathy and hypercalcemia remains unclear. On the one hand, alteration of electrolyte flux (Na^+ and Ca^{2+} increase) in the ventricular myocardium occurs before there is pathologic evidence of cardiomyopathy,[27] suggesting an early role in the drug-mediated disease process. On the other hand, Daniels et al.[28] have reported that, although high doses of calcium antagonists may protect against the cardiomyopathy produced by adriamycin, Bristow[3] has reported no protective effects of calcium antagonists when they were administered in doses that could be tolerated for several months. The inability of tolerable doses of calcium antagonists to prevent adriamycin cardiomyopathy therefore suggests that an abnormality of calcium translocation may not be a primary pathogenetic mechanism.[3]

One of the more well-established theories of anthracycline-mediated cardiotoxicity involves the drug-dependent production of free radicals and their effect on cardiac membranes. Aspects of this theory were recently fully reviewed by Myers,[1] Bristow,[3] and Pratt and Ruddon[5] and hence only a brief summary of this theory will be presented. It is now clear that many anthracyclines undergo reductive conversion in vivo and in vitro to semiquinone radicals that in turn, rapidly react with molecular oxygen to produce the superoxide radical.[1] Superoxide radicals are known to participate in a variety of reactions leading to the generation of hydroxy radicals and hydrogen peroxide with concomitant membrane damage and/or death of the cells in which this occurs.

The specificity of this theory resides in the fact that, although normal mammalian cells appear to possess elaborate defenses against oxidative radical attack,[29] cardiac tissue is less capable of preventing or reducing this type of histopathologic damage. Doroshow et al.[30] have pointed out that cardiac tissue is acatalasemic. In addition, there is an anthracycline-mediated drop in glutathione peroxidase activity, as noted by Reves and Marusic.[31] Since both catalase and glutathione peroxidase activities play essential roles in preventing membrane lipid peroxidation by catabolizing hydrogen peroxide and lipid hydroperoxides, the absence or reduction of normal levels of these activities in cardiac tissue may permit adverse membrane alteration and destruction, leading in turn to either reduced myocyte functioning or cellular death.

The reduction in anthracycline-mediated histopathologic damage produced by pretreatment with the free radical scavengers vitamin E,[17] cysteamine,[32] and N-acetylcysteine[33] has added support to the importance of free radical membrane damage as an important etiologic factor in anthracycline cardiotoxicity. This protective effect, however, could not be reproduced by several laboratories[3,34,35] and has led Bristow[3] to conclude that, although this does not rule out free radical-initiated and lipid peroxidation-mediated cardiac tissue damage in chronic anthracycline cardiotoxicity, it is evidence against it. Bristow further suggests that the high-dose, subacute anthracycline cardiotoxicity described in mice by Myers et al.[17] against which vitamin E is effective, may be mediated by a different mechanism than the chronic cardiac type of damage against which vitamin E treatment appears ineffective.

Adriamycin may also interfere with lipid transport. Experimental adriamycin cardiotoxicity has been reportedly improved by therapy with carnitine which is a vitamin responsible for the transport of activated fatty acid (acyl-CoA) from outside the inner mitochondrial membrane to within the mitochondria.[36] The importance of this theory of drug-mediated cardiotoxicity is questionable, however, since other investigators have reported little if any effect of carnitine in either preventing or reducing anthracycline cardiomyopathy.[37]

A final series of recently described phenomena may help to explain the production of cardiac failure produced by anthracyclines. Burns and Dow[38] have noted that daunorubicin-induced membrane damage in cardiac tissue is associated with the production of irreversible work failure without any significant decline in normal concentrations of either ATP or creatine phosphate. These authors suggested that the explanation for anthracycline cardiotoxicity must lie beyond either a direct inhibition of ATP degradation (e.g., ATPase activity) or of inhibition of the synthesis of either actin or myosin. Our laboratory has recently demonstrated[39] that this uncoupling of energy production from energy utilization may be explained by an anthracycline-mediated inhibition of the binding of creatine phosphokinase to the inner mitochondrial membrane. Whether this inhibition of enzyme-membrane binding, and hence the transfer of high-energy phosphate groups from ATP to creatine,[40] is due to direct drug binding to inner membrane cardiolipin or membrane lipid peroxidative damage is at present unclear. Nevertheless, drug binding to mitochondrial membrane has now been shown to produce both direct and indirect inhibition of key enzyme activities and/or function, the importance of which to the etiology of anthracycline cardiomyopathy remains to be further elucidated.

The multiple proposed mechanisms of action of anthracyclines with regard to the production of cardiomyopathic alterations readily point out the complex pharmacology of this class of drugs. Yet, the rational search for less cardiotoxic analogues of adriamycin and thus the eventual clinical utilization of anthracycline compounds with enhanced therapeutic indices depends on a much fuller understanding of the etiology of this drug-induced heart disease.

REFERENCES

1. Myers CE: In *Cancer Chemotherapy, Annual 2*, Pinedo HM (Ed), Elsevier North-Holland, New York, 1980, pp 66–83.
2. Bristow MR, Billingham ME, Minobe WA, et al.: *J Mol Cell Cardiol II (Suppl 1): 10*, 1979.
3. Bristow MR: In *Drug-Induced Heart Disease*, Bristow MR (Ed), Elsevier North-Holland, New York, 1980, pp 192–215.
4. Rosenhoff SH, Brooks E, Bostick F, Young RC: *Biochem Pharmacol 24, 1898*, 1975.
5. Pratt WB, Ruddon RW: In *The Anticancer Drugs*, Oxford University Press, New York, 1979, pp 148–194.
6. Flalkoff H, Goodman MF, Seraydarian MW: *Cancer Res 39: 1321*, 1979.
7. Lampidis TJ, Moreno G, Salec C, et al.: *J Mol Cell Cardiol 11: 415*, 1979.
8. Billingham ME, Mason JW, Bristow MR, Daniels JR: Anthracycline cardiomyopathy monitored by morphologic changes. *Cancer Treat Rep 62: 865*, 1978.
9. Lefrak EA, Pitha J, Rosenheim S, Gottieb JA: *Cancer 32: 302*, 1973.
10. DuVernay VH, Mong S, Crooke ST: In *Anthracyclines: Current Status and New Developments*. Crooke ST, Reich SD (Eds), Academic Press, New York, 1980, pp 61–123.
11. Levey GS, Levey BA, Ruiz E, Lehotay DC: *Cancer Res 11: 591*, 1979.
12. Gosalvez M, Van Rossum GDV, Blanco MF: *Cancer Res 39, 257*, 1979.
13. Solomonson LP, Halabrin PR: *Cancer Res 41: 570*, 1981.

14. Taylor D, Hochstein P: *J Cell Biol 83: MU2117, 1979.*

15. Ferrero ME, Ferrero E, Gaja G, Bernelli-Zazzera A: *Biochem Pharmacol 25: 125, 1976.*

16. Yasumi M, Minaga T, Nakamura K, *et al.*: *Biochem Biophys Res Commun 93: 631, 1980.*

17. Myers CE, McGuire WP, Liss RH, *et al.*: Adriamycin: The role of lipid peroxidation in cardiac toxicity and tumor response. *Science 197: 165, 1977.*

18. Dhalla NS, Fedelesova M, Toffler I: *Can J Biochem 49: 1202, 1971.*

19. Bernt E, Bergmeyer HU: In *Methods of Enzymatic Analysis*, Vol. 2. Bergmeyer HU (Ed), Academic Press, New York, 1974, pp 624–627.

20. Duarte-Karim M, Ruysschaert JM, Hildebrand J: *Biochem Biophys Res Commun 71: 658, 1976.*

21. Zanon PL, Lambertenghi-Deliliers G, Pozzoli EF, *et al.*: *Tumori 66: 27, 1980.*

22. Tritton TR, Murphee SA, Sartorelli AC: *Biochem Biohys Res Commun 84: 802, 1979.*

23. Olson HM, Young DM, Prieur DJ, *et al.*: *Am J Pathol 77: 439, 1974.*

24. Anghileri LJ: *Arzneim Forsch 27: 1177, 1977.*

25. Olson HM, Capen CC: *Lab Invest 37: 386, 1977.*

26. Moore L, Landon EJ, Coomey DA: *Biochem Med 18: 131, 1977.*

27. Billingham ME: In *Drug-Induced Heart Disease.* Bristow MR (Ed), Elsevier North-Holland, New York, 1980, pp 127–149.

28. Daniels JR, Billingham ME, Gelbart A, Bristow MR: *Circulation 54: 11–20, 1976.*

29. Chance B, Sies H, Boveris A: *Physiol Rev 59: 527, 1979.*

30. Doroshow JH, Locker GY, Myers CE: *J Clin Invest 65: 128, 1980.*

31. Revis NW, Marusic N: *J Mol Cell Cardiol 10: 945, 1978.*

32. Olson RD, MacDonald JS, Harbison, *et al.*: *Fed Proc 36: 303, 1977.*

33. Doroshow JH, Locker GY, Myers CE: *Proc Am Assoc Cancer Res 20: 1035, 1979.*

34. Breed JGS, Zimmerman ANE, Pinedo HM: *Cancer Res 40: 2033, 1980.*

35. Van Fleet JF, Ferrans VJ: *Cancer Treat Rep 64: 315, 1980.*

36. Opie LH, *Am Heart J 97: 375, 1979.*

37. Goldsmith MA, Suzuki Y, Ohnuma T, Holland JF: *Cancer Treat Rep 63: 558, 1979.*

38. Burns JH, Dow JW: *J Mol Cell Cardiol 12: 95, 1980.*

39. Newman RA, Hacker MP, Fagan MA: *Biochem Pharmacol 31: 109–111, 1982.*

40. Bessman SP, Geiger PJ: Transport of energy in muscle: The phosphorylcreatine shuttle. *Science 211: 448, 1981.*

Part III

The Trigon of Host, Tumor, and Anthracyclines

CHAPTER 9

The Trigon of Host, Tumor, and Anthracycline in Single Drug and Combination Therapy

A. Goldin, A. Rahman, A. M. Casazza, F. Giuliani, A. Di Marco, N. O. Kaplan, and P. S. Schein

With the known anthracycline derivatives and in the selection of potentially useful analogues, whether employed alone or in combination, consideration should be given to factors pertaining to the host–tumor relationship that may contribute to the achievement of maximum therapeutic effectiveness. New drugs may be investigated in detail and comparisons made on the basis of the total potential in terms of the possibility of manipulating the host–tumor relationship successfully. Such considerations must take into account both the ability to improve therapeutic response and to avoid unfavorable limiting toxicities to the host. This is particularly important for the anthracyclines where there are already several known derivatives with demonstrated clinical activity.

Division of Cancer Treatment, National Cancer Institute, Bethesda, Maryland; Division of Medical Oncology School of Medicine, Vincent T. Lombardi Cancer Research Center, Georgetown University Hospital, Washington, D.C.; Division of Experimental Oncology B Istituto Nazionale per lo Studio e la Cura dei Tumori, Milan, Italy; Farmitalia Carlo Erba, Milan, Italy; Department of Chemistry and the Cancer Center, University of California at San Diego, La Jolla, California

Factors Pertaining to the Host–Tumor Relationship in the Selection of New Anthracyclines

DRUG DOSAGE

Adriamycin (doxorubicin) differs from the parent compound daunomycin (daunorubicin) in the substitution of a hydroxyl group for a hydrogen atom in the acetyl radical of the aglycone moiety.[1-3] On similar schedules, such as treatment on a single day (day 1) and daily treatment (days 1–9), adriamycin was moderately but consistently more effective than daunomycin at a series of tolerated dose levels in increasing the survival time of mice with leukemia L1210.[4,5] But for each drug, with further increase in dosage, the toxicity of the drugs for the host became limiting and the survival time diminished. Nevertheless, lesser limiting toxicity for the host, such as myelosuppression and cardiotoxicity, and/or greater antitumor specificity, is implicit in the demonstration of greater therapeutic effectiveness of adriamycin in a system that employs survival time as the response parameter.

Myelosuppression and cardiotoxicity have represented two cardinal limitations in the therapy with anthracyclines, and any reduction in these toxicities, with retention of antitumor effect, would create interest in a new anthracycline derivative.

THE TUMOR SYSTEM EMPLOYED

The extent of difference in therapeutic response may be dependent upon the tumor system employed for comparison. In the P388 leukemia system, adriamycin was considerably more effective than daunomycin when the drugs were administered every 6 hours for a single day, on day 1 following leukemic inoculation. It was also more effective than daunomycin, but not as extensively, when treatment was every 3 hours on day 1 only.[4,5]

HOST–TUMOR HISTOCOMPATIBILITY

That the host may have a profound effect on the therapeutic outcome is illustrated in a study in which a comparison was made of the effectiveness of adriamycin in the therapy of leukemia L1210 in histocompatible $CD2F_1$ mice and BALB/c mice differing only in multiple minor histocompatibility loci. Adriamycin was highly effective and resulted in a number of cures over a series of dosages in the BALB/c-bearing L1210 mice, whereas the drug was only moderately effective in the treatment of tumorous syngenic animals.[6-8]

SCHEDULE OF THERAPY

The schedule of therapy may have an important effect on the therapeutic outcome. Adriamycin was more effective than daunomycin over a wide range of dosage schedules in increasing the life-span of mice with leukemia L1210. In addition, adriamycin treatment resulted in a somewhat greater number of long-term survivors.[4,5] Although in this and in other experiments, multiple I.P. treatment with adriamycin for a single day was the optimal schedule for leukemia L1210; in other experiments schedule dependency was not as evident.[9] Scheduling characteristics of new analogues could be examined to determine whether limiting toxicities can be reduced without proportionate loss of therapeutic effect.

ROUTE OF DRUG ADMINISTRATION

The route of administration may also have a marked effect on drug activity. For both adriamycin and daunomycin there was a marked loss in therapeutic effectiveness in the treatment of leukemia L1210 when the drugs were administered orally, indicating that there is a lack of absorption of the drugs from the gastrointestinal tract.[4] Where an anthracycline derivative is capable of eliciting a therapeutic response when administered orally, this could result in an advantage in therapy.

BODY BURDEN OF TUMOR CELLS

The body burden of tumor cells may also influence the therapeutic activity of antitumor drugs. With leukemia P388, B16 melanoma, Lewis lung carcinoma, and Ridgway osteogenic sarcoma, delay in treatment until the disease had become more advanced resulted in a decrease in therapeutic response.[9,10] An anthracycline derivative that retains its activity or exerts more extensive activity against advanced disease could provide an advantage in therapy.

EXTENT OF SPECTRUM OF ACTIVITY IN EXPERIMENTAL TUMOR SYSTEMS

It has been indicated both on the basis of retrospective and prospective analyses that high and broad-spectrum activity in a variety of tumor systems may predict at least minimal clinical activity for one or more human tumors.[11,12] Such high and broad-spectrum activity has been demonstrated for Adriamycin.[9,13] Activity has been observed against experimental lymphomas and leukemias,[1,4,14-16] myeloma,[1] sarcomas,[1,10,17,18] carcinomas,[1,19-22] and melanoma.[20,23] A new anthracycline derivative with more extensive activity in the same spectrum of tumors or with activity in tumor systems in which adriamycin has been ineffective would create interest for further development.

CROSS-RESISTANCE CHARACTERISTICS

Interest in an anthracycline derivative could result if it were active, or at least showed partial activity, against a tumor that had become resistant to adriamycin or daunomycin; or if the spectrum of cross-resistance were different from that observed with adriamycin or daunomycin.

The cross-resistance characteristics of a resistant subline of leukemia P388 has been reported.[9,24,25] It showed only partial resistance to cinerubin A, which has structural similarities to adriamycin.[9,24] However, cinerubin A appears to exert a similar degree of cardiotoxicity to that observed with adriamycin, which would tend to preclude serious clinical interest.[24] The adriamycin-resistant P388 subline exhibited cross-resistance to a number of anthracyclines including, daunomycin, rubidazone, carminomycin, and adriamycin-14-octanoate.[24]

Lack of cross-resistance characteristics for a new anthracycline derivative could make it highly attractive for use against adriamycin-resistant tumors.

POTENTIAL OF SELECTIVE DELIVERY SYSTEMS

Attempts have been made to improve the therapeutic effectiveness of anthracycline derivatives by alteration of the selective delivery characteristics. Complexes of anthracyclines with DNA have been employed to obtain selectivity by means of phagocytic engulfing of the complex by the tumor cells and the release of the anthracycline in the tumor cells by the lysosomes.[26] An anthracycline analogue attached in such a DNA complex that would be more active than either adriamycin alone or the adriamycin-DNA complex would provide a derivative of interest for further development.

The incorporation of antitumor agents into liposomes may alter the *in vivo* distribution of the entrapped agent and improve its distribution to the target site. Adriamycin was entrapped in positive liposomes composed of phosphatidylcholine, cholesterol, and stearyl amine and in negative liposomes composed of phosphatidylcholine, cholesterol, and phosphatidylserine. The amount of adriamycin captured in positive liposomes was 35% of the total input dose and about 55% in negative liposomes. Adriamycin entrapped in positive liposomes has been demonstrated to decrease the *in vivo* uptake of the drug into cardiac tissue of DBA/2 mice as compared with free drug or drug entrapped in negative liposomes (Table 1).[27] Cardiotoxicity studies in mice have shown reduced acute cardiac damage when adriamycin is administered entrapped in positively charged liposomes. The entrapped positive liposomes retain their antitumor activity against P388 leukemia and Lewis lung carcinoma (Table 1). Recently[28] chronic cardiotoxicity studies of adriamycin, free and entrapped in positive and negative liposomes, were performed in DBA/2 mice at a total dose of 28 mg/kg I.V. The mean quantitative and qualitative scores for lesions of cardiac damage were 2.7 and 2.23 for free adriamycin and adriamycin entrapped in negative liposomes, respectively. However, the mean score for the group of mice treated with positive liposomes was reduced substantially, the value being 1.20. Such reduction of acute and chronic cardiotoxicity by adriamycin entrapped in positive liposomes without loss of antitumor activity could provide an advantage for therapy. Investigations of selective delivery could be of value not only with respect to improvement of the therapeutic response to adriamycin but also in relation to the potential of new anthracycline derivatives.

ACTIVITY IN COMBINATION CHEMOTHERAPY

There is great interest in the utilization of combinations of drugs, based on the successes in the clinic. Adriamycin has

Table 1. Effect of Liposomal Entrapment of Adiamycin on Concentration × Time (CXT) Values and Activity in P388 Leukemia and Lewis Lung Carcinoma

	CXT (μg/hr/g^{-1})[a]				P388[b] ILS, %	Lewis Lung[c] Tumor Size in % of Controls at 16 Days
	Heart	Lung	Liver	Spleen		
Free doxorubicin	55.2	60.7	88.6	101.7	130	52
Doxorubicin entrapped in negative liposomes	83.4	59.6	211.2	174.3	112	66
Doxorubicin entrapped in positive liposomes	40.1	104.3	408.2	394.7	112	54

[a]Tissue levels of adriamycin fluorescent equivalents were determined in DBA/2 mice after I.V. injection of adriamycin (4 mg/kg) as free drug or drug entrapped in liposomes. CXT values calculated for the period from 5 minutes to 24 hours.
[b]Mice given I.P. injections of 10^5 cells and 24 hours later free or liposome-entrapped adriamycin (4 mg/kg) was administered I.P.
[c]Lewis lung carcinoma implanted S.C. Adriamycin (4 mg/kg) was administered I.V. as free or liposome-entrapped drug on days 8, 10, and 12 after tumor inoculation.
See Rahman et al.[27]

demonstrated broad-spectrum therapeutic synergism in experimental tumor systems when employed in combination with anti-metabolites, alkylating agents, and other types of drugs.[9,10,20,23] A difference in the spectrum of therapeutic synergism, or greater therapeutic activity than that observed with adriamycin in combination therapy, whether the drugs are employed concomitantly or in sequence, would make a new derivative of interest.

If a new anthracycline derivative demonstrated therapeutic synergism when employed in combination with adriamycin or daunomycin, there would be the suggestion of a difference in biochemical or pharmacologic action, which would focus attention on the new derivative.

In the treatment of leukemia L1210 therapeutic synergism was obtained with the combinations of adriamycin plus ICRF-159 and adriamycin plus cyclophosphamide.[23] With both combinations, there was a reduction in the optimal dosage of adriamycin. Such reduction in optimal dosage may help in the avoidance of limiting cardiac toxicity. In the utilization of a new anthracycline derivative it could be determined whether there was any further advantage in combination therapy in regard to dosage reduction.

SURGICAL ENCHANCEMENT OF DRUG EFFECT

The combination of surgery plus anthracycline may impove therapeutic response, and this should be taken into account in the investigation of new antitumor agents. Schabel et al.[29] in surgical adjuvant chemotherapy of subcutaneously implanted mammary adenocarcinoma demonstrated that administration of adriamycin prior to or subsequent to surgery was more effective than surgery alone or adriamycin alone in increasing the survival time and number of long-term survivors. In another study by Giuliani et al.,[30] surgery plus the combination of Adriamycin and cyclophosphamide was demonstrated to be highly effective in the reduction of lung metastases of the MS-2 sarcoma in BALB/c mice. In the bioassay for lung metastases following therapy, the number of takes was reduced from 100 to 6.6%.[30]

DRUG ENHANCEMENT WITH RADIATION

The combination of adriamycin plus radiation may result in therapeutic enhancement. In one experiment, treatment of the Ridgway osteogenic sarcoma with Adriamycin in combination with ^{60}Co gamma irradiation was more effective in increasing survival time than treatment with drug alone or radiation alone at comparable doses.[31]

IMMUNOSUPPRESSIVE CHARACTERISTICS

Adriamycin has proven to be less immunosuppressive than daunomycin. In one study in which there was pretreatment with daunomycin or adriamycin of animals with virus-induced Moloney sarcoma, there was progressive growth of tumor following pretreatment with daunomycin, whereas at equitoxic doses of adriamycin the tumor grew initially and then regressed in similarity to the untreated controls.[17] In another experiment in which treatment was administered following MSV (M)-induced tumors, the tumor grew progressively in all of the daunomycin-treated animals, whereas with adriamycin treatment there was marked initial regression of tumor in similarity to the controls.[17] Diminished immunosuppression for a new anthracycline derivative could make the compound of interest.

Factors Pertaining to the Host-Tumor Relationship with New Doxorubicin Derivatives Modified in the 4' Position of the Amino Sugar

In view of the previous discussion it is of interest to examine some of the data on new adriamycin derivatives. Three adriamycin derivatives modified in position 4' of the amino sugar, namely, 4'-epi-doxorubicin, 4'-deoxy-doxorubicin, and 4'-0-methyl-doxorubicin[32-35] are of current interest. Among themselves, and relative to adriamycin, the analogues exhibit individual differences as well as similarities in their pharmacological and therapeutic characteristics.

4'-Deoxy-doxorubicin and 4'-0-methyl-doxorubicin exerted acute toxicity (LD_{50}) at lower dosage than adriamycin.[35] With 4'-epi-doxorubicin, the LD_{50} was equivalent or somewhat higher than that of adriamycin.

The minimal cumulative cardiotoxic doses for 4'-deoxy-doxorubicin and 4'-0-methyl-doxorubicin were higher than that for adriamycin, although the optimal cumulative antitumor doses in the treatment of Gross leukemia were lower. The ratio of minimal cumulative cardiotoxic to optimal cumulative antitumor doses was more than twofold higher for 4'-deoxy-doxorubicin and 4'-0-methyl-doxorubicin as compared with adriamycin. This is suggestive of a greater therapeutic margin of safety (therapeutic ratio) in the use of the analogues where cardiotoxicity may be limiting. The ratio of cardiotoxic to tumor doses was slightly higher for the 4'-epi-doxorubicin as compared with adriamycin.[35]

The cardiac toxicity of 4'-deoxy-doxorubicin in rabbits was markedly reduced as compared with that observed with adriamycin. The cardiac toxicity for 4'-epi-doxorubicin was moderately reduced.[35]

In the treatment of a series of human colorectal tumors heterotransplanted in athymic (nude) mice, adriamycin was essentially ineffective, whereas 4'-deoxy-doxorubicin and 4'-0-methyl-doxorubicin showed definitive activity against a number of the tumors.[36]

In summary of the characteristics of 4'-deoxy-doxorubicin relative to adriamycin: 1) 4'-deoxy-doxorubicin had higher potency (1.5–2 times; active at lower doses).[35] 2) The activity was equal in the treatment of mouse leukemias and also against advanced C3H mammary carcinoma.[35,37] 3) It had higher effectiveness against human colon adenocarcinomas in nude mice and against colon 38 in mice.[36,37] 4) It had reduced cardiotoxicity in rabbits and in mice.[35,37] 5) Differences in pharmacokinetic properties are indicated by more rapid elimination from the heart, but not from tumor in mice.[38]

Thus, there are sufficient significant differences between 4'-deoxy-doxorubicin and adriamycin to warrant interest in development for this compound. Similarly, there are significant differences between 4'-o-methyl-doxorubicin and 4'-epi-doxorubicin, relative to adriamycin, which makes the adriamycin derivatives modified in position 4' of the amino sugar of special interest for detailed investigation, to determine the factors that may further improve their therapeutic effectiveness, with diminished limiting toxicity for the host. The potential of such drugs will be realized with detailed investigations of their activity, taking into account the trigon of host, tumor, and anthracycline derivative in single drug, drug combination, and combined modality therapy.

REFERENCES

1. Di Marco A, Gaetani M, Scarpinato B: Adriamycin (NSC 123, 127), a new antibiotic with antitumor activity. *Cancer Chemother Rep 53: 33–37, 1969.*
2. Aracamone F, Cassinelli C, Di Marco A, *et al.*: British Patent Application, Farmitalia Research Laboratories, 1969.
3. Arcamone F, Cassinelli G, Fantini G, *et al.*: Adriamycin, 14-hydroxydaunomycin, a new antitumor antibiotic from S. peucetius var. caesius. *Biotechnol Bioeng 11: 1101–1110, 1969.*
4. Sandberg JS, Howsden FL, Di Marco A, *et al.*: Comparison of the antileukemic effect in mice of adriamycin (NSC-123127) with daunomycin (NSC-82151). *Cancer Chemother Rep 54: 1–7, 1970.*
5. Goldin A: Some factors influencing the chemotherapeutic effectiveness of adriamycin. In: *Proceedings of the International Symposium on Adriamycin.* (Carter, SK, Di Marco A, Ghione M, *et al*, (Eds), Springer-Verlag, New York, 1972, pp 64–74.
6. Riccardi C, Kline I, Peruzzi L, *et al.*: Increased efficiency of antineoplastic agents in presence of antitumor immune responses in mice. Proceedings of the Fifth Pharmacology-Toxicology Symposium, 1977, p 56.
7. Goldin A, Nicolin A, and Bonmassar E: Interrelationship between chemotherapy and immunotherapy in the treatment of disseminated disease. *Recent Results Cancer Res 68: 458–464, 1979.*
8. Riccardi C, Bartocci A, Puccetti P, *et al.*: Combined effects of antineoplastic agents and antilymphoma allograft reactions. *Eur J Cancer 16: 23–33, 1980.*
9. Goldin A, and Johnson RK: Experimental tumor activity of adriamycin (NSC-123127). *Cancer Chemother Rep 6: 137–145, 1975.*
10. Schabel FM, Jr: Animal models as predictive systems. In: *Cancer Chemotherapy — Fundamental Concepts and Recent Advances*. Yearbook Medical Publishers, Chicago, 1975, pp 323–355.

11. Goldin A, Serpick AA, Mantel, N: A commentary. Experimental screening procedures and clinical predictability value. *Cancer Chemother Rep 50: 173–218, 1966.*
12. Goldin A, Venditti JM, Macdonald JS, *et al.*: Current results of the screening program at the Division of Cancer Treatment, National Cancer Institute. *Eur J Cancer 17: 129–142, 1981.*
13. Di Marco A: Adriamycin (NSC-123127). Mode and mechanism of action. *Cancer Chemother Rep 6: 91–106, 1975.*
14. Schwartz HS, and Grindey GB: Adriamycin and daunorubicin: A comparison of antitumor activities and tissue uptake in mice following immunosuppression. *Cancer Res 33: 1837–1844, 1973.*
15. Di Marco A, Casazza AM, Dasdia T, *et al.*: Cytotoxic, antiviral, and antitumor activity of some derivatives of daunomycin (NSC-82151). *Cancer Chemother Rep 57: 269–274, 1973.*
16. Frei E, III, Schabel FM, Jr, and Goldin A: Comparative chemotherapy of AKR lymphoma and human hematological neoplasia. *Cancer Res 34: 184–193, 1974.*
17. Casazza AM, Di Marco A, and Di Cuonzo G: Interference of daunomycin and adriamycin on the growth and regression of murine sarcoma virus (Moloney) tumors in mice. *Cancer Res 31: 1971–1976, 1971.*
18. Hoshino A, Kato T, Amo H, *et al.*: Antitumor effects of adriamycin on Yoshida rat sarcoma and L1210 mouse leukemia-cross-resistance and combination chemotherapy. In: *Proceedings of the International Symposium on Adriamycin.* Carter SK, Di Marco A, Ghione M, *et al.* (Eds), Springer-Verlag, New York, 1972, pp 75–89.
19. Di Marco A, Lenaz L, Csazza AM, *et al.*: Activity of adriamycin (NSC 123127) and daunomycin (NSC-82151) against mouse mammary carcinoma. *Cancer Chemother Rep 56: 153–161, 1972.*
20. Griswold DP, Laster WR, Jr, and Schabel FM, Jr: Therapeutic potentiation by adriamycin and 5-(3,3-dimethyl-1-triazeno)-imidazole-4-carboxamide) against B16 melanoma, C3H breast carcinoma, Lewis lung carcinoma and leukemia L1210. *Proc Am Assoc Cancer Res 14: 15, 1973.*
21. Keys L, Kende M, Johnson RK, *et al.*: Chemotherapeutic response of BALB/c mice with epithelial tumors (ET). *Fed Proc 33: 582, 1974.*
22. Ovejera AA: Growth characteristics and chemotherapeutic response of iv implanted Lewis lung carcinoma (LL). *Proc Am Assoc Cancer Research and ASCO 16: 109, 1975.*
23. Goldin A, and Johnson RK: Antitumor effects of adriamycin in comparison with related drugs and in combination chemotherapy. In: *Adriamycin Review.* Staquet M, Tagnon H, Kenis Y, *et al.* (Eds), European Press: Medikon, Ghent, Belgium, 1975, pp 37–54.
24. Johnson RK, Ovejera AA, and Goldin A: Activity of anthracyclines against an adriamycin (NSC-123127)-resistant subline of P388 leukemia with special emphasis on cinerubin A (NSC-18334). *Cancer Treat Rep 60: 99–102, 1976.*
25. Goldin A, and Johnson RK: Resistance to antitumor agents. In: *Recent Advances in Cancer Treat-*

ment. Tagnon HJ, and Staquet MJ, (Eds). Raven Press, New York, 1977, pp 155–169.

26. De Duve C, De Barsy T, Poole B, *et al.*: Lysosomotropic agents. *Biochem Pharmacol 23:* 2495–2531, 1974.

27. Rahman A, Kessler A, More N, *et al.*: Liposomal protection of adriamycin produced cardiotoxicity in mice. *Cancer Res 40: 1532–1537, 1980.*

28. Rahman A, White G, More N, *et al.*: Protection of chronic cardiotoxicity of adriamycin by liposomal delivery. *Proc Am Assoc Cancer Res 22: 269, 1981.*

29. Schabel FM, Jr, Griswold DP, Jr, Corbett TH, *et al.*: Recent studies with surgical adjuvant chemotherapy or immunotherapy of metastatic solid tumors of mice. In: *Adjuvant Therapy of Cancer II.* Jones SE, and Salmon SE (Eds), Grune & Stratton, New York, 1979, pp 3–17.

30. Giuliani F, Di Marco A, Casazza AM, *et al.*: Combination chemotherapy and surgical adjuvant chemotherapy on MS-2 sarcoma and lung metastases in mice. *Eur J Cancer 15: 715–723, 1979.*

31. Goldin A, Wodinsky I, Merker PC, *et al.*: Search for new radiation potentiators. *Int J Radiat Oncol Biol Phys 4: 23–35, 1978.*

32. Arcamone F, Penco S, Vigevani A, *et al.*: Synthesis and antitumor properties of new glycosides of daunomycinone and adriamycinone. *J Med Chem 18: 703–707, 1975.*

33. Arcamone F, Penco S, Redaelli S, *et al.*: Synthesis and antitumor activity of 4'-deoxydaunorubicin and 4'-deoxyadriamycin. *J Med Chem 19: 1424–1425, 1976.*

34. Cassinelli G, Ruggieri D, Arcamone F: Synthesis and antitumor activity of 4'-0-methyldaunorubicin, 4'-0-methyladriamycin and 4'-epi analogues. *J Med Chem 22: 121–123, 1979.*

35. Casazza AM, Di Marco A, Bonadonna G, *et al.*: Effects of modifications in position 4 of the chromophore or in position 4' of the amino sugar, on the antitumor activity and toxicity of daunorubicin and doxorubicin. In: *Anthracyclines: Current Status and New Developments.* Crooke ST, and Reich SD (Eds), Academic Press, New York, 1980, pp 403–430.

36. Giuliani FC, and Kaplan NO: New doxorubicin analogs active against doxorubicin-resistant colon tumor xenografts in the nude mouse. *Cancer Res 40: 4682–4687, 1980.*

37. Casazza AM, Bellini O, Savi G, *et al.*: Antitumor activity and cardiac toxicity of 4'-deoxydoxorubicin (4'-deoxydx) in mice. *Proc Am Assoc Cancer Res 22: 267, 1981.*

38. Formelli F, Fumagalli A, Giuliani F, *et al.*: Tissue distribution of doxorubicin (DX) and 4'-deoxydoxorubicin (4'-deoxydx) in nude and conventional mice bearing colon tumors. *Proc Am Assoc Cancer Res 22: 267, 1981.*

Part IV

Biochemical Pharmacology

CHAPTER 10

Mechanisms of Action of the Anthracycline Antibiotics

N. R. Bachur

In Chapter 8 Dr. Newman compiled a complete and extensive list of anthracycline antibiotic actions that have been related to the well-known anthracycline-induced cardiotoxicity. This accumulation of cardiotoxicity data serves to indicate to us that 1) the anthracycline antibiotics are involved in multiple actions, and 2) considering the mechanism of antitumor action of the anthracycline antibiotics, the relationship between cardiotoxicity and antitumor action is unclear. I will indicate several actions of the anthracycline antibiotics that may cause their antitumor action as well as their cardiotoxicity. Since we, as scientists, always seek a single "cause and effect" relationship, we may feel uncomfortable with too many causes and too few relationships. However, I will return to this point later.

As pharmacologists, our studies of drugs always bring us to scrutinize the molecular structure to understand how the molecule works. The clinically active anthracycline antibiotics have certain structural features common to all and apparently necessary for pharmacologic activity. These include 1) the tetracyclic planar three-ring system with the fourth ring saturated and nonplanar, 2) a quinone–hydroquinone system; 3) a glycosidic or aminoglycosidic moiety. Other features of the anthracycline antibiotic molecules may

vary considerably and may affect the pharmacokinetics and the pharmacodynamics of the agents, but other modifications seem to be less important to the principal actions of the antibiotics than the three just listed.

With the discovery of the antitumor activity of daunorubicin and adriamycin, astute scientists were quick to propose that the structure of these biotoxins would favor an interaction with DNA and a mechanism of action based on this interaction. Experimentation followed with clear and elegant data that daunorubicin and adriamycin bind to DNA, primarily through intercalative binding, but also by nonintercalative modes. After studying the mode of binding by x-ray crystallography, DNA pertubations, and atomic model fitting, the scientists have concluded that these antibiotics intercalate into double-stranded DNA with the planar ring system lying between stacked base pairs. The positively charged amino sugar protrudes from the coiled DNA and ionically binds to the negatively charged phosphate sugar esters of the main DNA chain. Such intercalative binding distorts the DNA helix and presumably interferes with the biochemical processing of the DNA.[1-3]

The biochemical effects of the anthracycline antibiotics have been examined by many investigators who have produced a consensus of biochemical evidence that the anthracycline antibiotics inhibit nucleic acid metabolism both rapidly and effectively. Experiments at various levels of biologic organization with tissues and iso-

Chief, Laboratory of Clinical Biochemistry, Baltimore Cancer Research Center, Division of Cancer Treatment, National Cancer Institute, National Institutes of Health, Baltimore, Maryland

lated cells show rapid uptake of adriamycin or daunorubicin into cells, followed by a rapidly increasing and almost complete inhibition of DNA and RNA synthesis, with DNA synthesis showing more complete inhibition than the RNA. When the biochemical machinery for nucleic acid synthesis and metabolism is dissected from the cell and assessed for anthracycline action, additional information becomes available. DNA polymerases from various sources yield to the anthracyclines dramatically. Adriamycin or daunorubicin at micromolar concentrations bind to the DNA template necessary for DNA polymerase action and inhibit the polymerase reaction very effectively and nearly completely. From studies with T_4 bacteriophage DNA polymerase, it appears that a three-membered, tight complex of DNA polymerase, antibiotic, and DNA is formed, which yields grudgingly to dissociation. Furthermore, when the DNA repair or editing 3'-exonuclease of T_4 bacteriophage is studied, the anthracycline antibiotics inhibit this important enzymatic sculptor of newly formed DNA. Other studies show that a number of functional characteristics of DNA are severely altered by the anthracycline binding to this life-critical macromolecule. All these inhibitory processes result from the tight and specific binding of the anthracycline antibiotic to DNA with a resultant *static* inhibition of the nucleic acid metabolism.

During the investigation of the action of the anthracycline antibiotic aclacinomycin A on cellular metabolism, Oki et al.[4] showed that this antibiotic had a different spectrum of action than adriamycin and daunorubicin. Aclacinomycin A preferentially inhibits RNA synthesis over DNA synthesis. Aclacinomycin A is representative of a group of anthracycline antibiotics that exhibit this preferential inhibitory action on nucleolar RNA synthesis and RNA synthesis over DNA synthesis.[5]

Despite the extensive investigations into the mechanism of action of the anthracycline antibiotics, several characteristics and actions of the antibiotics have not yielded to explanation by the static inhibition evidence. One such characteristic is the ability of these antibiotics to kill cells that are not undergoing cell division and the associated required DNA and RNA synthesis. Although cells in S phase are usually very sensitive to anthracycline antibiotics, experimental evidence shows that noncycling cells are also killed by the drugs. This is especially significant in the clear clinical effects of adriamycin on slow-growing solid tumors. Another action not explained by the static inhibition evidence is the clastogenic effect of the antibiotic. Chromosomes from cells pretreated with the antibiotics have severe deformation and damage compared to normal chromosomes. Similarly, the DNA isolated from cells pretreated with the anthracyclines shows an increasing pattern of breakage with increasing anthracycline antibiotic concentrations. All of these actions of DNA breakage cannot be accomplished by simply mixing DNA with the antibiotic. Something else is necessary.

We feel that the something else necessary to cause DNA destruction and possibly other actions by the anthracycline antibiotics is biologic activation of the antibiotic molecule. Evidence for biologic activation of the anthracycline molecule first appeared in metabolism studies of the anthracycline antibiotics in animals and human beings. These studies showed that one type of metabolite isolated from urine, bile, and tissues and produced in *in vitro* metabolism experiments was a 7-deoxyaglycone. Normally, in a hydrolytic reaction of the anthracycline glycosides, a 7-hydroxyaglycone is formed. Special reaction circumstances are required to form the 7-deoxyaglycone. These conditions are to have healthy microsomes; the electron donor, NADPH; the anthracycline antibiotics; and the absence of oxygen. If oxygen is included in the reaction, a reaction occurs involving the NADPH, microsomes, and the antibiotic, which causes the rapid consumption of the oxygen but no apparent change of the antibiotic. After all the oxygen in the reaction mixture is consumed, the antibiotic rapidly breaks at the glycosidic bond and yields the 7-deoxyaglycone.[6]

Detailed investigation of the reaction that yields 7-deoxyaglycones indicates that the NADPH functions as an electron donor for the single-electron reduction of the anthracycline antibiotic. This reduction occurs at the quinone region of the anthracycline molecule to yield the single-electron reduced antibiotic, the semiquinone, which is an unstable free radical form that is very reactive. As long as oxygen is available, no single-electron reduction of the antibiotic is apparent. But, this is misleading, for it is by a futile reduction process that the oxygen is consumed and converted into superoxide. Oxygen is a very avid acceptor of the free radical electron from the semiquinone anthracycline. When all the oxygen is consumed and converted to superoxide, then the semiquinone anthracycline antibiotics demonstrate their instability by undergoing reductive glycosidic cleavage to the 7-deoxyaglycones.

Recent studies show that the oxygen that participates in this single electron transfer reaction is responsible for DNA breakage. The superoxide produced may react directly with the DNA to cause cleavage or may react further to produce hydroxy radical or other activated molecules, which may cause the DNA breakage that has been observed in chemical and enzymatic systems.[7,8]

The enzymatic machinery in the microsomes has been dissected and shown that the flavoprotein NADPH cytochrome P-450 reductase is the enzyme responsible for transfer of the single electron from NADPH to the receptor anthracycline antibiotic quinone system. Other flavoproteins, such as xanthine oxidase, NADH cytochrome c reductase, and nitrate reduc-

tase also catalyze the oxygen consumption, the production of 7-deoxyaglycones, and the free radical production.[9] Widespread importance of flavoproteins in mammalian tissues suggests that the free radical activation of the anthracycline antibiotics probably occurs throughout the tissues. Certainly the isolation of 7-deoxyaglycones from many tissues of both animals and patients strengthens this position.

Since cell nuclei are the principal residence of the cellular DNA, and the nuclei are known to contain drug metabolizing flavoproteins such as NADPH cytochrome P-450 reductase, it is important to determine whether nuclei catalyze anthracycline antibiotic free radical formation. These experiments show that cell nuclei catalyze free radical production, superoxide production, and 7-deoxyaglycone production. Thus the very package that houses the DNA also contains the enzymes to produce the reactive free radical forms.[10] Microsomes for all tissues tested show catalytic activity for the activation process, although the specific activities vary. Therefore this reaction potential appears ubiquitous in mammalian tissues, although the range of reactivity is wide. All the anthracycline antibiotics tested show activation by the microsomal, nuclear, or appropriate flavoprotein system, but none show any significantly higher affinity or rate of free radical formation.

In a second consideration of the structure of the anthracycline antibiotics, it is clear why the tetracyclic ring system and the glycosidic moieties are essential to cytotoxic activity in tailoring the molecules to possess tight binding characteristics for the DNA structure. With the new observations related to the electron transfer characteristics and free radical formation of the anthracycline antibiotics, it becomes evident why the quinone–hydroquinone system may be necessary for activity of these agents. The combination of these structural characteristics — 1) the affinity of the anthracycline antibiotics to bind to DNA perhaps with more specificity than we are able to resolve at present, and 2) the ability of the antibiotic to be activated to and to generate the formation of additional reactive free radicals — led to the concept of the *"site-specific free radical"* for agents of this type.[11]

Although we as scientists continually seek the final common denominator or the single basic cause-and-effect relationship, it is possible that the anthracycline antibiotics do not possess a single mechanism of action; but possess numerous mechanisms of action. From the point of view of the *Streptomyces* working to develop the most potent and dependable toxin in its struggle against numerous and varied soil microorganisms, it makes good sense to produce a toxin that has multiple mechanisms of action. Such a toxin would be active against more types of opponent microognisms, and opponent microorganisms would suffer biochemical stress to self-induce resistance to more than one mechanism of action. From this perspective, it may be that anthracycline antibiotics have several modes of action at various levels in the cell: the nucleus, the cell membrane, and the cytoplasm. These modes may relate to the specific binding of the drug to such macromolecules as DNA, but also may relate to the activation of the drug metabolically to yield highly reactive free radicals. Such free radical production may involve oxygen as a destructive agent

in free radical transfer or may utilize other radical reactions. Clearly, the anthracycline antibiotics are very specifically tailored structures; and small modifications in structure lead to major differences in cytotoxicity, spectrum of action, and specificity of action. Until these very complex and extensive questions of the modes of action of the anthracycline antibiotics are answered and organized into a clear unified picture, I prefer to look upon the beautiful anthracycline molecules not as biochemical inhibitors with a single inhibitory action, but rather as molecules honed through eons of time to yield multiple effects in the living system.

REFERENCES

1. DiMarco A, Arcamone F: *Arzneim Forsch 25: 368*, 1975.
2. Waring M: *J Mol Biol 54: 247, 1970.*
3. Henry DW: Symposium, cancer chemotherapy. *Am Chem Soc 30: 15, 1976.*
4. Oki T, Matsuzawa Y, Yoshimoto A, Numata K, Kitamura I, Hori S, Takamatsu A, Umezawa H, Ishizuka M, Naganawa H, Suda H, Hamada M, Takeuchi T: *J Antibiot (Tokyo) 28: 830 1975.*
5. Crooke ST, Duvernay VH, Galvan L, Prestayko AW: *Mol Pharmacol 14: 290, 1978.*
6. Bachur NR, Gordon SL, Gee MV: *Mol Pharmacol 13: 901, 1977.*
7. *76: 765, 1977.*
8. Berlin V, Haseltine WA: *J Biol Chem 256: 4747,* (1981.
9. Pan SS, Bachur MR: *Mol Pharmacol 19: 184, 1981.*
10. Bachur NR, Friedman RD, Gee MV: *Proc Am Assoc Cancer Res 20: 128, 1979.*
11. Bachur NR, Gordon SL, Gee MV: *Cancer Res 38: 1745, 1978.*

CHAPTER 11

Structure–Activity Relationships

F. Arcamone

Following the development of daunorubicin and doxorubicin as useful drugs in the medical treatment of human tumors, studies aimed at the discovery of analogues endowed with higher efficacy and less side effects have been carried out in laboratories throughout the world. Therefore both the chemistry and the biochemistry of the anthracyclines have been actively investigated. Although important developments have been recorded in these fields, as deduced from the availability of new compounds now in the clinical stage and from the collection of a great amount of data concerning their mechanism of action, the complexity of the problems facing those involved in the aforesaid objective is clearly apparent from the literature. However, the biologic activity is a function of the structure of a drug, and the structure of a drug implies certain molecular properties that are the basis of its pharmacologic behavior.

In this account I shall therefore summarize results obtained in our laboratory on the effect of chemical modifications on antitumor activity and on molecular properties currently considered of relevance within this defined group of chemotherapeutic agents. We may classify the daunorubicin and doxorubicin analogues in five groups, namely: 1) simple derivatives of the biosynthetic glycosides, 2) compounds bearing modifications at the C-9 side chain, 3) semisynthetic glycosides of daunomycinone and adriamycinone, 4) compounds showing different substitution in the anthraquinone chromophore (rings B, C, D), and 5) compounds bearing modifications on ring A.

Simple derivatives of the biosynthetic glycosides include compounds of pharmacologic interest, such as doxorubicin esters, daunorubicin benzoylhydrazone, and N-trifluoroacetyldoxorubicin-14-valerate. For two of these derivatives the biotransformation to the parent compound in vivo has been demonstrated.

Compounds bearing modifications at the C-9 side chain may retain the antitumor activity in experimental mouse tumors, as was the case of daunorubicinol, doxorubicinol, 9-deacetyldaunorubicin, 9-deacetyl-9-hydroxymethyldaunorubicin, or they may exhibit a reduced activity, as occurred with the 14-aminodaunorubicins and the 13,14-epoxide analogue. The 9-deacetyl analogue is currently under preclinical evaluation at the National Cancer Institute in the United States as compound NSC 268708 because of its lower cardiotoxicity when compared with doxorubicin.

In our studies a great importance has been attributed to modifications of the carbohydrate moiety. This is because of the known dependence of cellular uptake processes (and therefore on tissue distribution and pharmacokinetics) and of enzyme–substrate specificity (and therefore on biotransformation reactions) on structure and stereochemistry in carbohydrate derivatives, and because the presence of daunosamine-related sugars in other antibiotics provided examples of variations compatible with high bioactivity.

Ricerca and Sviluppo Chimico, Farmitalia Carlo Erba, Milano, Italy

Within a range of stereochemically and structurally modified glycosides, a compound with the L-*arabino* configuration (4′-epidoxorubicin, I), in which the sugar moiety is the natural amino sugar L-acosamine, and a compound with a 4′-deoxy group and L-*threo* configuration (4′-deoxydoxorubicin, II), in which the sugar moiety is 4′-deoxydaunosamine (a new amino sugar), have been found to possess outstanding pharmacologic properties. As a matter of fact I is presently undergoing phase 2 clinical trials, and II is in advanced preclinical stage. Whereas the stereochemical variants with an axial amino group (L-*ribo* and L-*xylo*) and the 6′-hydroxylated analogues exhibited a reduced antitumor efficacy and/or potency, other analogues modified at C-4′ retained the biologic activity of the parent compounds. Among the latter, mention should be made of the 4′-O-methyl derivatives III and of the more recently synthesized 4′-C-methyl analogues. The compatibility of the C-4′ substitution, which is also exhibited by different biosynthetic anthracyclines with high bioactivity, is also shown in the disaccharide analogues 4-daunosaminyldaunorubicin, 4-α-acosaminyldaunorubicin, and 4′-(α-L-2-deoxyfucosyl)daunorubicin (Fig. 1).

Another important group of new analogues is the one resulting from totally synthetic aglycones with different substitutions on ring D. It appears that a wide variety of modifications in ring D substitution is compatible with bioactivity, the 4-demethoxy analogues IV and V being outstanding for their potency (compound IV is also active when administered orally and is now undergoing clinical trials in different centers) and antitutmor efficacy. On the other hand, substitution of one of the two hydroxyl groups at C-6 and C-11 with a methoxyl in the daunorubicin and carminomycin series resulted in a reduction of antitumor activity with respect to the parent drugs. However, the isolation of 11-deoxydoxorubicin from cultures of *Micromonospora peucetica* and the recent

synthesis of the corresponding 4-demethoxy analogue reported by Umezawa et al. have allowed the characterization of the 11-deoxy modification as a useful one, deserving further investigation.

With ring A modifications, we face a diversified reality. This ring bears the two asymmetric centers of the aglycone moiety, the C-7 center being of major importance, as it establishes the general symmetry of the molecule. As expected, the C-7(R) analogues are biologically inactive, whereas the inversion at C-9 as in 9-deacetyl-9-epidaunorubicin induces only a partial reduction of antitumor activity. Position 9 is important because the C-9 hydroxyl has been considered as involved in a 1,3 hydrogen bonding with the C-7 oxygen or, alternatively, as involved in an intermolecular hydrogen bonding to a purine residue in the minor groove of DNA. The finding that the 9-deoxy analogues still possess antitumor activity is of interest in this respect. However, the 9α-methoxy and 9α-methyl analogues do not exhibit antitumor properties in the mouse P388 test. Another modification of interest is the substitution at C-8 with a methoxyl or a methyl group, 8β-methoxydaunorubicin being comparable to daunorubicin in the P388 test. It is worth noting that a methoxyl group at the same position is present in steffimycin A. Loss of bioactivity was also found in the 10(S)-substituted analogue VI, whereas the 10(R) compound VII exhibited activity comparable to the parent in the P388 test, antitumor activity still being evident, but lower than in the doxorubicin-treated animals, in compound VIII. It should be noticed here that the stereochemistry at C-10 of the said 10(R) derivatives is the one also present in the biosynthetic anthracyclines bearing a carbomethoxy group at C-10. Finally, the importance of ring A spatial arrangement for the expression of bioactivity is shown by the complete loss of antitumor effect in analogues with a double bond at C-9, C-10, or in the cyclopropane analogue 9-

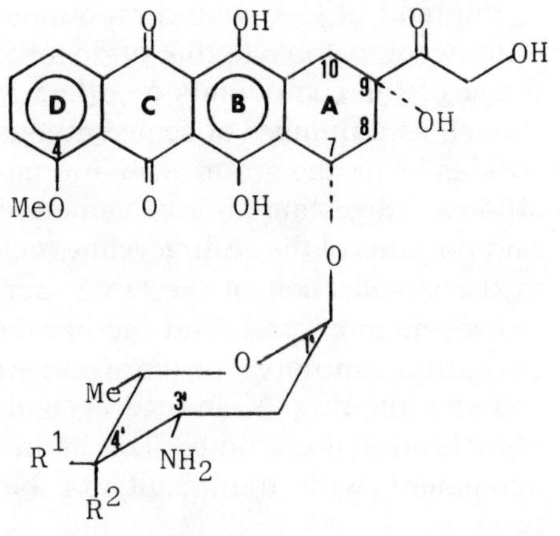

I :R^1= OH, R^2= H
II :R^1= R^2= H
III:R^1= N, R^2= OMe

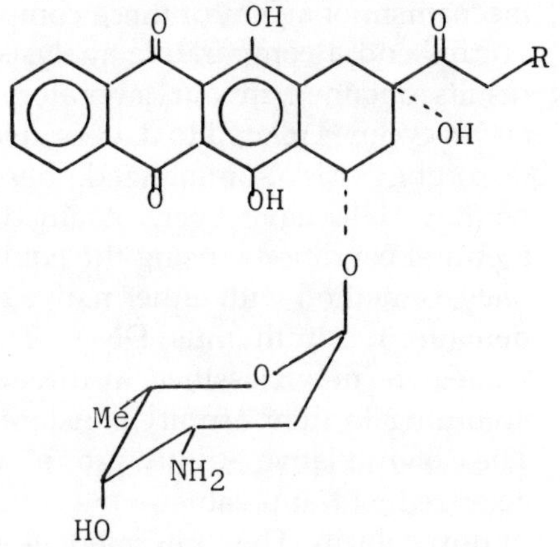

IV: R= H
V : R= OH

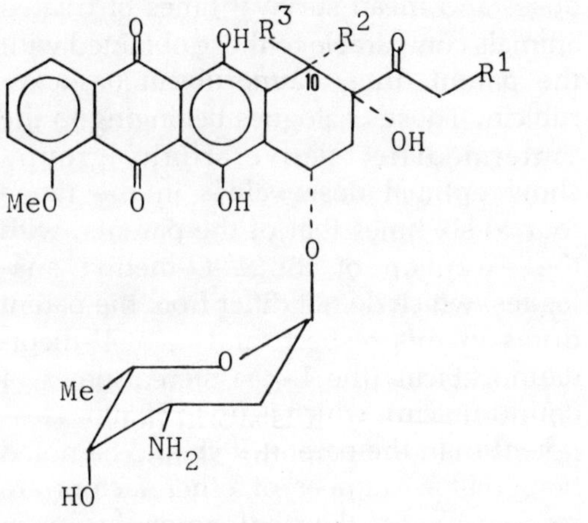

VI : R^1= R^3= H, R^2= OMe
VII : R^1= R^2= H, R^3= OMe
VIII: R^1= OH, R^2= H, R^3= OMe

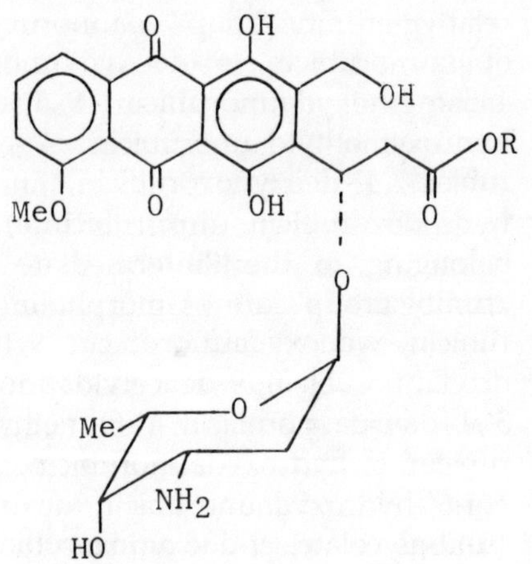

IX: R= H
X : R= Me

FIGURE 1. Stereochemically and structurally modified glycosides.

deoxy-9,10-methanodaunorubicin. Also, opening of the A ring to give IX and X appeared to be deleterious as far as the exhibition of antitumor activity was concerned.

A necessary step for the understanding of the structure–activity relationship is the correlation of structural and stereochemical features with molecular interactions of pharmacologic relevance and the correlation of the same with the biologic effects. It is obvious that the ability of antitumor anthracyclines to bind to native double-helical DNA is the first interaction that should be taken into consideration because of the current views concerning the mechanism of action of these compounds. To this end a comparative analysis of the results obtained in our laboratory on 27 anthracyclines related to daunorubicin and doxorubicin is summarized here. The binding data have been obtained under identical conditions, using the equilibrium dialysis method with either native or heat-denatured calf thymus DNA. The analogues are now classified in three groups according to their affinity constant Kapp. The "high relative affinity group" is characterized by Kapp values $\geq 80\%$ the value of doxorubicin. The "intermediate relative affinity group" is characterized by Kapp value in the range of 50–80% the value of doxorubicin. The "low relative affinity group" is characterized by Kapp values $< 50\%$ the value of doxorubicin. The following compounds belong to the "high relative affinity group": daunorubicin, 4'-epidaunorubicin, 4'-deoxydaunorubicin, 4-demethoxydaunorubicin, 9-deacetyl-9-hydroxymethyldaunorubicin, 4'-epidoxorubicin, 4'-deoxydoxorubicin, and 13-dihydrodoxorubicin (doxorubicinol). Those belonging to the "intermediate relative affinity group" are 14-morpholinodaunorubicin, 9-deoxydaunorubicin, 9,10-anhydrodaunorubicin, 9-deacetyldaunorubicin, 3',4'-diepidaunorubicin, 4'-O-methyldaunorubicin, 6'-hydroxydaunorubicin, 3',4'-diepi-6'-hydroxydaunorubicin, doxorubicin-14-O-glycolate, 9-deoxydoxorubicin, and 4'-O-methyldoxorubicin. Finally, included in the "low relative affinity group" are the following compounds: 3'-epidaunorubicin, 1',4'-diepidaunorubicin (a β-anomer), 4'-epi-4'-O-methyldaunorubicin, 9-deacetyl-9-epidaunorubicin, 4-demethoxy-7,9,1'-triepidaunorubicin [(7R), 9(R) β-anomer], doxorubicin-14-octanoate, 1'-epidoxorubicin (the β-anomer of doxorubicin), 3',4'-diepi-6'-hydroxydoxorubicin, and N-acetyldoxorubicin.

From these lists it appears clearly that the structural requirements for the high affinity toward DNA are rather strict. Only modifications in the C-9 side chain, in the D ring and at C-4' give compounds with affinity comparable to that of doxorubicin. Some of the compounds modified at C-9 as well as a number of semisynthetic glycosides fall in the group with intermediate affinity, suggesting an involvement of the said portions of the anthracycline molecule in the stabilization of the DNA complex. However, more profound modification of the sugar moiety, or configurational changes on ring A, induce a significant reduction of the affinity. This is in good agreement with the results of biologic tests.

An inspection of the antitumor activity in the mouse experimental leukemia of compounds just listed shows that those analogues belonging to the "high relative affinity group" display optimal (nontoxic) doses and mean survival times of treated animals comparable to those obtained with the parent drug, daunorubicin or doxorubicin. Those analogues belonging to the "intermediate relative affinity group" show optimal dose values in the range four to six times that of the parents, with the exception of the 4'-O-methyl analogues, which do not differ from the parent drugs in this respect, and of 3',4'-diepidaunorubicin (the L-$ribo$ stereoisomer of daunorubicin), which is up to 50 times less potent than the parent. It should be noted here that a number of other factors are responsible for the final expression of in $vivo$ activity, and, aside from potency, the efficacy of the optimal doses in terms of increase of survival is always comparable with that of the parents.

A different situation appears when the biologic activity of the compounds belonging to the "low relative affinity group" is considered. Clearly, this group includes compounds with measurable affinity, such as doxorubicin-14-octanoate, 4'-epi-4'-O-methyldaunorubicin and 9-deacetyl-9-epidaunorubicin (Kapp 20–25% of that shown by the parent drug) together with derivatives showing much lower affinity, such as N-acetyldoxorubicin. For this reason and for the complication due to metabolism, a wide variation in the bioactivity was found. Doxorubicin-14-octanoate was as active as the parent, but its transformation into doxorubicin *in vivo* is well established. 4'-epi-4'-*O*-methyldaunorubicin and 9-deacetyl-9-epidaunorubicin displayed still appreciable antitumor activity, but the optimal doses were at least six times those of daunorubicin. No activity was exhibited at the highest dose tested for 3'-epidaunorubicin and for the two β-anomers. *N*-acetyldoxorubicin was nearly as active as doxorubicin but at more than 100-fold dosage, suggesting also the possibility of a metabolic deacylation *in vivo*.

Lipophilicity is currently accepted as a parameter of drug activity and its relevance in the class of the antitumor anthracyclines has been checked by determining the "lipophilic index" (log K') by reverse-phase high pressure liquid chromatography, using a buffered (pH 7.0 tris, 30°) 35% mixture of acetonitrile and water as mobile phase, according to Yamada *et al.* The following log K' values were found: daunorubicin, 0.48; 4-demethoxydaunorubicin, 0.69; 3',4'-diepidaunorubicin, 0.77; doxorubicin, 0.016; 4'-epidoxorubicin, 0.14; 4'-*O*-methyldoxorubicin, 0.26; 4'-deoxydoxorubicin, 0.30; 4-demethoxydoxorubicin, 0.33. It appears that a wide variation exists in the lipophilic properties of bioactive anthracyclines, with a trend (if any) toward increased potency with lipophilicity in the doxorubicin series, and no effect on efficacy.

The question of what molecular property relates with the antitumor efficacy and spectrum in experimental animals and in the clinics is obviously complex, and the answer requires other types of information. One is that represented by the behavior of the drug in the animal body in respect to distribution, elimination, and metabolic fate. The availability of radio-labeled anthracyclines has now opened the way to qualitative and quantitative comparative analysis of related compounds. A recent study performed in rats in the author's laboratory has shown that [^{14}C]4'-epidoxorubicin differs considerably from [^{14}C]doxorubicin because of a significantly higher initial concentration in kidney, lung, and bone marrow, but lower in blood and, at later times, in heart tissue. In agreement with previous findings obtained by the use of the fluorescence assay method, a more rapid clearance of 4'-epidoxorubicin in comparison with doxorubicin has also been demonstrated. These results may be of help in order to explain the more favorable pharmacologic properties of the analogue.

If the affinity for the DNA receptor is a necessary condition, but not a determinant of optimal antitumor efficacy, other molecular interactions are responsible for it. In fact, the antitumor anthracyclines show binding interactions with proteins, such as plasma proteins, nonhistone proteins from rat liver chromatin, spectrin, tubulin, actin, and heavy meromyosin, human erythrocyte ghost membranes. In addition to proteins, other macromolecular species show binding interactions with the antitumor anthracyclines. These include rat liver RNA, f2 phage RNA, yeast transfer RNA, heparin and chondroitin sulfate, cardiolipin, phospholipid constituents of Ca^{2+} transport system, liposomes, and negatively charged phospholipids.

In conclusion, until contrary evidence is produced, the following statements can be made: 1) Modifications of daunorubicin and doxorubicin molecules at C-4', on ring D substitution and at C-9 side chain, afford analogues with high antitumor activity; 2) other modifications have induced reduction of efficacy and/or potency; the stereochemistry at C-7 and C-1', and the conformation of ring A are strict requirements for bioactivity; 3) affinity for DNA correlates with potency; 4) wide variations in lipophilicity have a small, if any, effect on potency, but not on efficacy; 5) pharmacologic properties, including distribution, kinetics, and metabolism, are responsible for optimal antitumor activity and other molecular interactions are probably involved.

BIBLIOGRAPHY

Aracamone F: Daunomycin and related antibiotics. In *Topics in Antibiotic Chemistry*, Vol. 2, Sammes PG (Ed). Ellis Horwood, Chichester, 1978, pp 100–239.

Arcamone F: *The Development of New Antitumor Anthracyclines*. Medicinal Chemistry Series, Vol. 16, Academic Press, New York, 1980, pp 1–40.

Arcamone F: *Doxorubicin*. Medicinal Chemistry Series, Vol. 17. de Stevens G (Ed). Academic Press, New York, 1981.

Arlandini E, Vigevani A, and Arcamone F: Interaction of new derivatives of daunorubicin and adriamycin with DNA. *Farmaco [Sci] 32: 315–223, 1977.*

Arlandini E, Vigevani A, Arcamone F: Interaction of new derivatives of daunorubicin and doxorubicin with DNA. Part II. *Farmaco [Sci] 35: 65–78, 1980.*

Goormachtigh E, Chatelain P, Caspers J, Ruysschaert JM: Evidence of a specific complex between adriamycin and negatively-charged phospholipids. *Biochim Biophys Acta 597: 1–14, 1980.*

Karczmar GS, Tritton TR: The interaction of adriamycin with small unilamellar vescicle liposomes. A fluorescence study. *Biochim Biophys Acta 557: 306–319, 1979.*

Neidle S: Interactions of daunomycin and related antibiotics with biological receptors. In: *Topics in Antibiotic Chemistry*, Vol. 2. Sammes PG (Ed). Ellis Horwood, Chichester, 1978, pp 240–278.

Quigley GJ, Wang AHJ, Ughetto G, Van Der Marel G, Van Boom JH, Rich A: Molecular structure of an anticancer drug-DNA complex: Daunomycin plus d(CpGpTpApCpG). *Proc Natl Acad Sci USA 77: 7204–7208, 1980.*

Shafer RH: Spectroscopic studies of the interaction of daunomycin with transfer RNA. *Biochem Pharmacol 26: 1729–1734, 1977.*

Sinha BK, Chignell CF: Interaction of antitumor drugs with human erythrocyte ghost membranes and mastocytoma P 815: A spin label study. *Biochem Biophys Res Commun 86: 1051–1057, 1979.*

Umezawa H, Takahashi Y, Naganawa H, Tatsuta K, Takeuchi T: Synthesis of 4-demethoxy-11-deoxy-analogs of daunomycin and adriamycin. *J Antibiot (Tokyo) 33: 1581–1585, 1980.*

Will J, Splitter G, Lalich J, Dennis S, Dennis W: *Adriamycin Cardiotoxicity: A Comparison with 9-Desacetyl Daunorubicin Hydrochloride* (NSC Number 268708). National Technical Information Service, Springfield, Va., 1980.

Yamada T, Tsuji A, Miyamoto E, Kubo O: Novel method for determination of partition coefficients of penicillins and cephalosporins by high-pressure liquid chromatography. *J Pharm Sci 66: 747–749, 1977.*

Zunino F, Casazza AM, Pratesi G, Formelli F, Di Marco A: Effect of the methylation of aglycone hydroxyl groups on the biological and biochemical properties of daunorubicin. *Biochem Pharmacol 30: 1856–1858, 1981.*

CHAPTER 12

Studies on the Cellular Pharmacology of Daunorubicin and Doxorubicin in Experimental Systems and Human Leukemia

C. Peterson[a], C. Paul[b], and G. Gahrton[b]

Clinical pharmacology studies during the last few years have revealed large interindividual variations in the absorption, distribution, metabolism, and excretion of many drugs.[12] By monitoring the plasma concentrations of cardiac glycosides and antiepileptics, for example, at steady state, it is most often possible to find out an individual dosage schedule so that the patient will achieve therapeutic effect without serious adverse side reactions.

In cancer chemotherapy, we may in the future come into a situation where more therapeutic benefit can be achieved by individualizing the therapy with existing drugs than by introducing new drugs. However, in order successfully to individualize the therapy we must have a better knowledge of the factors that determine the therapeutic and toxic responses of the individual patient and the interindividual variability of these factors.

The effect of a certain chemotherapeutic agent on those cells that are targets for the therapeutic and toxic effects of the drug is dependent on the concentration and subcellular localization of the drug and its active metabolites in the cells as well as on the specific toxic effects of the active substances on cellular processes. The specific inhibitory effect of daunorubicin (DNR) and doxorubicin (DOX) on the DNA and RNA synthesis in cultured cells is very similar.[2] Yet, there is a clear difference in the clinical activity spectra between the drugs, DOX being much more effective against solid tumors, whereas both drugs are active against leukemia.[4] Since most cancer chemotherapeutic drugs, such as the anthracyclines, are administered intermittently, no steady-state concentrations are obtained in plasma, which makes it difficult to draw conclusions on the concentrations in the target cells from plasma concentration data. However, leukemic patients offer a unique opportunity to study the pharmacokinetics of cancer chemotherapeutics in a compartment that can be regarded as a target for the cytostatic therapy, namely, the circulating leukemic cells.

During the last few years, we have studied the cellular pharmacology of DNR and DOX in various experimental systems as well as in human leukemia.

In Vitro Studies

We have compared the accumulation of DNR and DOX in various cell types. The drugs were assayed by total fluorescence, since, under *in vitro* conditions, very little metabolism occurs as determined by high pressure liquid chromatography (HPLC).[9] Cell counts and drug concentrations were selected so that the cellular uptake did not

[a]Department of Pharmacology, Karolinska Institute, S-104 01 Stockholm, Sweden
[b]Section of Clinical Hematology, Department of Medicine, Huddinge Hospital, S-141 86 Huddinge, Sweden

reduce the drug concentration in the incubation medium by more than 30%. Assuming uniform intracellular distribution, the ratios between the intracellular and the extracellular concentrations have been calculated (Table 1). The volume of the fibroblasts and the leukemic cells was calculated from the protein content, assuming that 1 mg of cell protein corresponds to a cell volume of 5 μl.[14] The value used for the volume of human red blood cells was 90 μm^3/cell. Since the chicken red blood cells contained twice as much hemoglobin as the human cells, a volume of 180 μm^3/cell has been used in the calculations. The results show that there is an extensive accumulation of DNR and DOX in nucleated cells, but not in human red blood cells.

Subcellular fractionation studies have shown that both DNR and DOX are stored in nuclei and lysosomes of cultured rat fibroblasts,[6] whereas in human leukemic cells the drugs are stored in nuclei only.[7] The nuclear trapping can easily be explained by the high affinity of the drugs for DNA. In the lysosomes the drugs are probably stored in protonated form as a result of the acid milieu.[10] The reason for the difference in subcellular localization of DNR and DOX between rat fibroblasts and human leukemic cells is at present not clear but may be attributed to differences in nuclear binding capacity or lysosomal volume or intralysosomal pH.

Table 1 also shows that the N-acetyl derivatives of DNR and DOX accumulate much less than the parent compounds in rat fibroblasts. Subcellular fractionation of the cells showed that these derivatives are neither trapped in nuclei nor in lysosomes,[10] indicating that the amino group of the sugar moiety is of great importance for both trapping mechanisms. The cytotoxicity of the N-acetyl derivatives is also much weaker than of the parent compounds.[15]

In spite of the very high intracellular accumulation of DNR and DOX, evidence from various experimental systems have been presented for an active efflux mechanism of anthracyclines across the plasma membrane.[3,5,9,10] By studying the effect of various incubation conditions, e.g., pH and metabolic inhibitors on drug accumulation in rat fibroblasts, we could explain the difference in cellular accumulation and subcellular distribution between DNR and DOX by a "leak and pump" model.[9,10] According to this hypothesis, drug influx occurs as passive diffusion of nonionized drug. Since DNR is more lipophilic than DOX, the diffusion of DNR will be faster. Because of the active efflux mechanism, the concentration of both drugs in the cell sap will be very low, but it will be higher for DNR than for DOX. Equilibration with the storage compartments in the nuclei and in the lysosomes will lead to an extensive intracellular drug accumulation. A schematic picture of the hypothesis is shown in Figure 1. Results from experimental systems indicate that development of anthracycline-resistant cell lines is accompanied by an enhanced activity of the active efflux system.[5,13]

Table 1. Calculated Ratios Between the Intracellular and Extracellular Concentrations of DNR and DOX During *in Vitro* Incubations at Steady State

Cells	DNR	DOX	N-Acetyl-DNR	N-Acetyl-DOX
Rat fibroblasts in culture, 17.5 μM, 5 ml medium/mg cell protein	800	150	15	5
Human red blood cells, 40 μM, 3 $\times$ 10^7 cells/ml	17	13		
Chicken red blood cells, 20 μM, 3 $\times$ 10^6 cells/ml	1100	540		
Human leukemic cells, 1.75 μM, 10^6 cells/ml	1500	560		

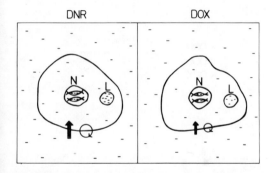

DNR   DOX

FIGURE 1. Schematic drawing of the "leak and pump" model for the cellular accumulation of anthracyclines. The drugs enter the cells by diffusion, DNR faster than DOX due to its higher lipophilicity. Intracellular drug is either trapped in nuclei (N) or lysosomes (L) or extruded across the plasma membrane by an active efflux mechanism.

Human red blood cells contain neither nuclei nor lysosomes, but yet the intracellular concentration of DNR and DOX at steady state markedly exceeded the concentration in the incubation medium. The N-acetyl derivatives also reached higher concentrations intracellularly than in the incubation medium in spite of the fact that the drugs are neither stored in nuclei nor in lysosomes. These observations may be explained by the lipid solubility of the drugs probably leading to enrichment in the cell membranes. This view is supported by observations of hemolysis at incubation with higher drug concentrations. In this respect, the red blood cells are more sensitive to DNR than to DOX, which is in accordance with the concentration ratios reached.

In Vivo Studies

During treatment of patients with acute nonlymphoblastic leukemia, we have compared the pharmacokinetics of DNR and DOX in plasma and in leukemic cells.[7] The drugs and their main metabolites were separated by HPLC in a straight-phase system with fluorometric detection as described elsewhere.[8] The plasma pharmocokinetic results are summarized in Table 2. The distribution volume of both drugs are extremely large, indicating a pronounced tissue affinity. There is also a large interindividual variation.

We have previously found that the plasma concentrations of DNR and its reduced metabolite, daunorubicinol, provide little information on the concentrations in the leukemic cells, which are targets for the therapy.[8] Figure 2 shows the concentrations of DNR, DOX, and their metabolites in leukemic cells from patient III (male, 56 years old) obtained during one treatment course with DNR and another with DOX some time later. Blood samples were collected during and after the drug infusions. Leukemic cells were immediately isolated and drug determination performed as described before.[8] At the start of the DOX course, no remaining drug could be found in plasma or leukemic cells. Also in vivo, there is an extensive intracellular accumulation of DNR and DOX. The peak concentration is higher for DNR. The ratios between the intracellular concentrations and the plasma concentrations at the end of the infusions can be calculated as previously described to 165 for DNR and 30 for DOX. Recent results on the toxicity of DNR on granulocyte-macro-

Table 2. Plasma Pharmacokinetic Parameters in Leukemic Patients Receiving DNR or DOX, 1.5 mg/kg Body Weight

Patient	Clearance $(1 \times h^{-1} \times kg^{-1})$	Vd $(1/kg)$
DNR Treatment		
I	2.00	53.8
II	0.86	52.8
III	1.16	48.3
IV	4.58	30.0
V	1.98	20.0
Mean values	2.12	41.0
DOX Treatment		
III	1.27	54.5
IX	1.02	20.4
X	1.29	26.6
Mean values	1.19	33.8

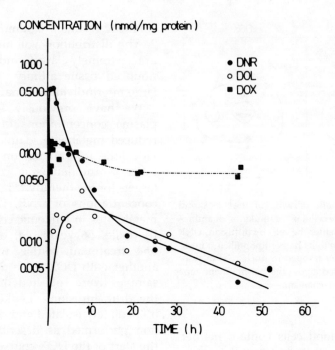

FIGURE 2.   Concentrations of DNR, DOX, and their metabolites in leukemic cells from peripheral blood of patient III isolated during one treatment course with DNR and another with DOX some time later.

phage stem cells from NMRI mice as assayed by their colony-forming ability in semisolid agar show that, at similar intracellular exposure doses, DNR is more toxic when present at a higher concentration for a shorter time as compared to a lower concentration for a longer time.[1] This indicates that the high peak concentration obtained for DNR may be of value for killing leukemic cells. On the other hand, DOX is retained much longer than DNR in the leukemic cells. This can be explained by the higher affinity of DOX for DNA[11] and may be of value for killing slowly growing solid tumor cells.

In plasma the concentration of daunorubicinol exceeds that of DNR already at the end of the infusions,[8] whereas the intracellular appearance of daunorubicinol is much slower. No metabolite of DOX could be found intracellularly.

Conclusions

There is an extensive intracellular accumulation of DNR and DOX in nucleated cells *in vitro* as well as *in vivo*. The accumulation of DNR is always higher than of DOX. This difference can be explained by a "leak and pump" model based on the higher lipophilicity of DNR. During treatment of leukemic patients, plasma concentrations on the drugs and their metabolites provide little information on the concentrations in the leukemic cells, which are targets for the therapy. Intracellularly, DNR reaches a higher peak concentration, whereas DOX is retained much longer. This difference in intracellular concentration pattern between DNR and DOX may very well explain the difference in clinical activity spectrum between these drugs. The high peak concentration obtained for

DNR is probably of importance for killing the leukemic cells, whereas the sustained intracellular concentration observed for DOX may be necessary in order to kill more slowly growing solid tumor cells.

REFERENCES

1. Andersson B, Beran M, Tribukait B, Peterson C: Significance of cellular pharmacokinetics for the cytotoxic effects of daunorubicin. *Cancer Res 42: 178–183, 1982.*
2. Bachur NR, Steele M, Meriwether WD, Hildebrand RC: Cellular pharmacodynamics of several anthracycline antibiotics. *J Med Chem 19: 651–654, 1976.*
3. Danö K: Active outward transport of daunomycin in resistant Ehrlich ascites tumor cells. *Biochim Biophys Acta 323: 466–483, 1973.*
4. Davis HL, Davis TE: Daunorubicin and adriamycin in cancer treatment: An analysis of their roles and limitations. *Cancer Treat Rep 63: 809–815, 1979.*
5. Inaba M, Kobayashi H, Sakurai Y, Johnson RK: Active efflux of daunorubicin and adriamycin in sensitive and resistant sublines of P388 leukemia. *Cancer Res 39: 2200–2203, 1979.*
6. Noël G, Peterson C, Trouet A, Tulkens P: Uptake and subcellular localization of daunorubicin and adriamycin in cultured fibroblasts. *Eur J Cancer 14: 363–368, 1978.*
7. Paul C: Anthracycline cytostatics in acute leukemia. Clinical and experimental studies with special reference to cellular pharmacology. Thesis, Karolinska Insitute, Stockholm, 1981.
8. Paul C, Baurain R, Gahrton G, Peterson C: Determination of daunorubicin and its main metabolites in plasma, urine and leukaemic cells in patients with acute myeloblastic leukaemia. *Cancer Lett 9:263–269, 1980.*
9. Peterson C, Baurain R, Trouet A: The mechanism for cellular uptake, storage and release of daunorubicin. *Biochem Pharmacol 29: 1687–1692, 1980.*
10. Peterson C, Trouet A: Transport and storage of daunorubicin and doxorubicin in cultured fibroblasts. *Cancer Res 38: 4645–4649, 1978.*
11. Schneider Y-J, Baurain R, Zenebergh A, Trouet A: DNA-binding parameters of daunorubicin and doxorubicin in the conditions used for studying the interaction of anthracycline–DNA complexes with cells in vitro. *Cancer Chemother Pharmacol 2: 7–10, 1979.*
12. Sjöqvist F, Borgå O, Orme MLE: Fundamentals of clinical pharmacology. In *Drug Treatment Principles and Practice of Clinical Pharmacology and Therapeutics.* 2nd ed. Avery GS (Ed), Churchill Livingstone, Edinburgh, 1980, pp 1–61.
13. Skovsgaard T: Mechanisms of resistance to daunorubicin in Ehrlich ascites tumor cells. *Cancer Res 38: 1785–1791, 1978.*
14. Tulkens P, Trouet A: Uptake and intracellular localization of streptomycin in the lysosomes of cultured fibroblasts. *Arch Int Physiol Biochim 80: 623–624, 1972.*
15. Yamamoto K, Acton EM, Henry DW: Antitumor activity of some derivatives of daunorubicin at the amino and methyl ketone functions. *J Med Chem 15: 872–875, 1972.*

CHAPTER 13

Intracellular Distribution of Anthracycline Antibiotics

N. R. Bachur

Occasionally, the study of the intracellular localization or distribution of a substance, such as a drug, leads to an understanding of the action or function of the substance. In the case of the anthracycline antibiotics, this appeared to be true until recently.

Adriamycin and daunorubicin are wonderful drugs to study, since they are not only brightly colored and produce brightly colored solutions, but they also fluoresce an intense orange-red color. The fluorescence property results from the highly conjugated anthraquinone ring system. Whereas many biologic molecules fluoresce, the anthraquinones have a unique type of fluorescence when compared to the fluorescent substances in mammalian tissues. No naturally occurring substances in mammals excite at 470 nm and emit at 550–580 nm as do the anthracycline antibiotics. This physical charactertistic of the molecules is very useful in the study of the biochemical and cellular pharmacology of the drugs. Since the fluorescence is an inseparable characteristic of the intact anthraquinone moiety, this property is used for the study of drug interactions and perturbations and for identification, characterization, and quantification of the drugs and of their metabolites. It was this property of fluorescence that Silverstini et al.[1] utilized to show that HeLa cells in-

cubated in tissue culture with daunorubicin concentrated the drug fluorescence in the nuclear structures. As an additional verification, these investigators utilized tritiated daunorubicin, which they localized through its radioactivity in the cell nucleus.

In efforts to determine the cellular disposition of adriamycin and daunorubicin in vivo, experiments were conducted with hamsters administered intravenous drug. Frozen sections of heart, liver, lung, and kidney revealed a rapid cellular uptake of both drugs and the principal concentration of the drug in the cellular nuclei.[2] For 15 minutes after administration, the nuclear drug fluorescence grew to a maximum. During this time, faint cytoplasmic fluorescence was visible in kidney tubular cells, but this cytoplasmic fluorescence disappeared after 15 minutes. Whereas the nuclei in all the tissues remained fluorescent for at least 60 minutes, there was no apparent redistribution of fluorescence evident. Since the anthracycline antibiotics have been shown to bind to numerous biologic macromolecules, it would seem reasonable to expect to see more cytoplasmic fluorescence. However, only occasional fluorescent granules are seen in the cytoplasm of some anthracycline-containing cells.

Although the cytofluorescence studies were carried out with intact cells and tissues in order to prevent drug redistribution when tissues are disassembled, Noel et al.[3] have studied the cellular uptake and distribution of adriamycin and daunorubicin in rat fibroblasts that are

Chief, Laboratory of Clinical Biochemistry, Baltimore Cancer Research Program, Division of Cancer Treatment, National Cancer Institute, National Institutes of Health, Baltimore, Maryland

assayed after cellular disassembly and isopycnic centrifugational isolation of the cellular components. Distribution of the adriamycin and daunorubicin between nuclear and cytoplasmic components from the rat fibroblasts indicated that between 30 and 40% of the intracellular adriamycin was cytoplasmic, whereas 70 to 80% of the daunorubicin was cytoplasmic. The remainder of the daunorubicin and adriamycin fluorescence was determined to be nuclear. When these authors fractionated the rat fibroblasts further and isolated the fractions by isopycnic centrifugation, postnuclear components were identified by marker enzymes; cytochrome c oxidase with mitochondria; NADH cytochrome c reductase with endoplasmic reticulum, 5'-nucleotidase with plasma membrane; and N-acetyl-β-glucosaminidase from lysosomes. There was strong association of daunorubicin fluorescence with the N-acetyl-β-glucosaminidase, which is the marker for lysosomes. Control experiments indicated that no redistribution of the drug occurred during the homogenization process. From these experiments, the conclusions are that most of the daunorubicin and a considerable proportion of adriamycin are localized in the cell cytoplasm, primarily in lysosomes. The studies, of course, differ from what has been observed by direct fluorescence inspection and by radioactive tracer. However, they bring to mind the question of the validity of any of these studies in terms of assessing intracellular distribution.

All localization studies had been done with adriamycin and daunorubicin until Krishan and his coworkers[4] studied the localization of the anthracycline analogue AD-32. AD-32 retains the intense fluorescence of the anthracycline family that easily remains an intracellular marker of its localization. When taken up by cells from tissue culture, AD-32 showed a negative type of distribution compared to daunorubicin or adriamycin. That is, the intense fluorescence of the drug is observed only in the cytoplasmic regions, revealing a black area for nuclei. This corresponded well to the in vitro observations that AD-32 did not appear to interact very effectively with isolated DNA.

In view of these conflicting data and disarray of understanding of the intracellular distribution of anthracyclines, we designed a series of experiments to assess the localization of a number of anthracycline analogues that were available through the Drug Development Program of the National Cancer Institute and that had numerous useful substitutions on the molecular structures. We selected a number of these to test their localization in cultured cells and also to determine the interaction of their fluorescence with DNA, RNA, or isolated L1210 nuclei. The cells that were used to assess these characteristics were L1210 murine leukemia cells, two strains of P388 murine leukemia, L929 mouse fibroblasts, and freshly isolated human neutrophils from peripheral venous blood. All of these cell types handled the drug cytofluorescence localization identically. The nuclear localized drugs again were daunorubicin and adriamycin, both of the N,N-dimethyl-substituted analogues of daunorubicin and adriamycin, and 4'-epidaunorubicin (Table 1).

Cytoplasmic drugs are by far the most numerous, and these gave almost exclusively cytoplasmic fluorescence with dark areas where the nuclei are localized. There were some cytoplasmic particles or inclusions that also showed intense fluorescence with some cytoplasmic drugs. A few of the agents appeared to distribute equally between nuclear and cytoplasmic compartments.

When the structures of the numerous analogues are compared and related to their cytoplasmic distribution, one clear correlation appeared. The methoxy group at carbon-4 of the anthraquinone system is critical for nuclear localization. The absence of the methoxy group in carminomycin or 4'-demethoxydaunorubicin is the

Table 1.   Intracellular Localization of
Anthracycline Antibiotics

Nuclear

Daunorubicin; adriamycin; *N,N*-dimethyldaunoru-
bicin; *N,N*-dimethyladriamycin; 4'-epidaunorubicin

Cytoplasmic

N-acetyldaunorubicin; *N,N*-dibenzyldaunorubicin;
3',4'-diacetyldeaminodaunorubicin; 4-demethoxy-
daunorubicin; carminomycin; marcellomycin;
musettamycin; aclacinomycin A; nogalomycin;
nogamycin; 7-dis-*O*-methylnogarol, and 7-con-*O*-
methylnogarol

Both

3'-Deaminodaunorubicin, *N*-formyladriamycin,
13-aminodaunorubicin

only difference between these cytoplasmic
localized compounds and the nuclear localized daunorubicin. Other modifications in
the anthraquinone structure may change
intracellular localization. For instance
modification at position 9 or the carbonyl
moiety at carbon-13 yield cytoplasmically
localized analogues of both adriamycin
and daunorubicin. In addition, modifications of the sugar moiety influence the
drug localization. Whereas *N,N*-dimeth-
ylation of the daunosamine amino group
or the inversion of the hydroxy group at
carbon-4' do not change the nuclear localization, larger substituents or charge modifications give analogues that are cytoplasmically localized.

A major criticism for the use of cytofluorescence has been that the fluorescent
drugs themselves are subject to fluorescence quenching when they bind to the
DNA of the nucleus; and therefore the absence of nuclear flourescence may not be a
valid critique. This is a reasonable criticism, which also points out the fact that,
although many of these drugs do not appear to bind to DNA, they cause rapid and
highly effective inhibition of DNA synthesis in cells and in *in vitro* systems. It is
interesting that anthracycline antibiotics,
such as carminomycin and marcellomycin,
that express cytoplasmic fluorescence are
accumulated avidly by isolated L1210 nu-

clei and retain the ability to inhibit DNA
synthesis. When the quenching of the
anthracycline fluorescence by DNA, RNA,
or isolated L1210 nuclei is examined, it is
clear that the addition of DNA to the drug
solutions and nuclei produces a rapid
quench of the drug fluorescence, which
varies with the compound.

In view of the complexities of measuring
intracellular fluorescence of drugs, I suggest that the cytofluorescence technique be
utilized as an experimental system. Some
of the factors that influence the intracellular
drug flourescence are 1) concentrating effect by subcellular components, 2) quenching of flourescence by binding to macromolecules, 3) enhancement of fluorescence
by solubilization in organic phases, and
4) quenching of flourescence by adsorption. It is reasonable to question data that
show contradictions. How does a drug
that does not appear to enter the cell
nucleus inhibit nucleic acid synthesis at
the replication level? Obviously, the inter-
relationships between flourescence localization and drug action need to be studied
further.

In an effort to understand more of drug
localization in subcellular systems, we
began the study of the anthracycline drugs
and cellular and macromolecular interaction in collaboration with Dr. Michel
Robert and Dr. Van Moudrianachis of the
Johns Hopkins University. The studies involve the use of chironomid, a midge.
These insects have salivary glands with
large nuclei that can be examined very
easily by flourescence microscopy and
show the localization and uptake of anthracycline drugs. Our studies with the
chironomous salivary gland show that
N,N-dimethyldaunorubicin, daunorubicin,
and adriamycin have a nuclear localization, whereas aclacinomycin A and carminomycin are primarily cytoplasmic.
These data support our previous findings.
However, the other important and interesting characteristic of the chironomous
salivary gland is that the nuclei can be iso-

lated from the cells by careful micromanipulation, and these nuclei contain giant chromosomes. The entire chromosomal structure is visible by light microscopy and can be activated by various chemical and biochemical maneuvers. In ongoing studies Dr. Robert has shown that the anthracycline agents bind to the polytene chromosomes to yield very beautiful fluorescence patterns, with specific degrees of banding. In addition, agents that normally do not enter the nucleus as determined by the cytofluorescence studies, such as 7-*O*-methylnogarol, show binding to the isolated giant polytene chromosomes and associated nucleolus.

I think that after the years of investigations of the intracellular localization studies of the anthracycline agents, it would best be stated that anthracycline antibiotics enter cells very rapidly and appear to bind and localize in various areas. Certainly, there appears to be clear indication that some bind to nuclear DNA and some are localized in subcompartments, such as lysosomes. It is unclear why a significant number of the agents do not appear to show flourescence in the nuclei, whereas they produce very intense biochemical effects on nuclear metabolism. It may be that only a small amount of the drug, not enough to be seen by flourescence, is needed to accomplish these biochemical effects in the nuclei. Since radioactive analogues are not available, the localization of the analogues through radioactive tracer has not been possible except in the case of tritiated daunorubicin. Perhaps in future studies we will pinpoint the specific site of action of the few anthracycline molecules that enter a cell and immobilize its life process.

ACKNOWLEDGMENTS

I would like to thank my collaborators in this work, Dr. Michel Robert and Dr. Merrill Egorin. I also thank the Foundation Simone et Cino Del Duca and others for the support of this symposium and Professor Mathé for his invitation.

REFERENCES

1. Silverstini R, Gambarucci C, Dasdia T: *Tumori 56:* 137, 1970.
2. Egorin MJ, Hildebrand RC, Cimino EF, Bachur NR: *Cancer Res 34:* 2243, 1974.
3. Noel G, Trouet A, Zenebergh A, Tulkus P: *EORTC International Symposium Adriamycin Review.* Staquet M, et al. (Eds), European Press Medikon, Ghent, Belgium, 1975, p 99.
4. Krishan A, Israel M, Modest EJ, Frei E: *Cancer Res 36:* 2114, 1976.
5. Egorin MJ, Clawson RE, Cohen JL, Ross LA, Bachur NR: *Cancer Res 40:* 4669, 1980.

CHAPTER 14

Comparative Uptake of Adriamycin, Daunorubicin, and Aclacinomycin-A in Sensitive and Resistant Friend Leukemia Cells

H. Tapiero, A. Fourcade, and M. Bennoun

Abstract

Based on the fluorescence properties of adriamycin (ADM), daunorubicin (DNR), and aclacinomycin A (ACM), uptake in sensitive and resistant Friend leukemia cells (FLC) was studied with the aid of the fluorescence activated cell sorter (FACS II) and by high pressure liquid chromatography (HPLC). It was shown that uptake, which is a very rapid process, was temperature dependent and was not hindered by sodium azide treatment.

The intracellular drug was mainly distributed in the nuclei. Incorporation into isolated nuclei was not temperature dependent nor hindered by sodium azide. We assumed therefore that incorporation across the plasma membrane is a passive process related to the composition and to the dynamic structure of the cell surface membrane.

Friend leukemia cell variants resistant to adriamycin (ADM-RFLC) and to daunorubicin (DNR-RFLC) were developed. The rate of uptake of ADM and DNR across the plasma membrane of these two cells variants was lower than in sensitive cells.

Although these cells were cross-resistant to both ADM and DNR, cell volume monitored by light scattering measurements and fluorescence intensity were distributed differently according to the resistant cell variant.

The rate of uptake of ACM across the plasma membrane of ADM-RFLC and DNR-RFLC was the same as in sensitive cells.

We suggest therefore that resistance is the consequence of changes induced in the plasma membrane components. These changes may be different according to the drug that is used.

Adriamycin (ADM), daunorubicin (DNR), and aclacinomycin A (ACM) are glycosidic anthracycline anticancer antibiotics[1-5] with bifunctional molecules containing a hydrophobic and a hydrophilic region. The hydrophobic region is composed of a resonating ring system introducing an intrinsic fluorescent property to the molecule. When this molecule is excited with an appropriate light wavelength, a fluorescence signal is obtained. By comparison with ADM and DNR, the structure of ACM is characterized by an ethyl group at C-9 instead of the acetyl or the hydroxyl acetyl group, the methoxy carbamyl group at C-10, and the hexopyranoses (rhodosamine, 2-deoxyfucose, and cinerulose) attached via glycosidic linkage at C-7. It was observed that ADM and DNR, when incor-

Département de Pharmacologie Cellulaire et Moléculaire et de Pharmacocinétique, Unité Simone et Cino Del Duca de Pharmacologie Humaine des Cancers, and, Institut de Cancérologie et d'Immunogénétique (INSERM U-50), Hôpital Paul-Brousse, Villejuif Cédex, France

porated into cells, were mainly distributed in nuclei.[6,7] Whereas ACM was classified by some authors as nonnucleophilic,[8,9] this classification will not be supported by the present study. Since the cytotoxic effect was correlated to an interaction with DNA altering the DNA-dependent DNA and RNA polymerase activities,[10-14] cellular uptake could be a decisive factor for the biologic and therapeutic effect of drugs belonging to this group. The exact mode of cellular uptake[15-19] and the mechanism by which this uptake could be altered *in vitro* and *in vivo* are not known.[20-22] The possibility that changes in the dynamic structural organization of the cell surface occurring in the development of cell resistance cannot be excluded. The present study was undertaken to determine the rate of incorporation of ADM, DNR, and ACM into sensitive and resistant cells.

Materials and Methods

CELL CULTURE

Friend leukemia cells (FLC) were derived from a clone of Friend virus-transformed cells 745A. Cells were grown in modified Eagle's spinner medium lacking calcium and containing 10 mM sodium phosphate and nonessential amino acids (Gibco). Medium was supplemented with 10% fetal calf serum (Gibco lot K 3862015) and antibiotics. All cell cultures were incubated at 37°C in a CO_2 incubator. Cell densities were determined by repeated cell counts using an hemacytometer, and cell viability was measured by counting the cells excluding 0.1% trypan blue.

The highly resistant cell variants, resistant to adriamycin (ADM-RFLC) and daunorubicin (DNR-RFLC), were derived from FLC 745A by continuous exposure to increasing concentrations of each drug over a period of 9 months and maintained at 1 μg/ml of ADM and DNR for 3 months. The resistant cell variants were then transferred for more than 70 passages without a

drug. Under these conditions, resistance was still maintained.

CHEMICALS

All chemicals were of analytical grade. Aclacinomycin A and adriamycin (doxorubicin hydrochloride) were kindly provided by the Roger Bellon Laboratory (Paris, France) and daunorubicin (daunorubicin hydrochloride) by Rhône-Poulenc (Paris, France).

CONDITION OF ADM AND DNR EXPOSURE AND MEASUREMENTS OF FLUORESCENCE INTENSITY

Unless otherwise noted, samples of 1×10^7 cells in 1 ml fresh growth medium were incubated with different concentrations of ADM and DNR. After an incubation period of 60 minutes at a given drug concentration and an appropriate temperature, labeled cells were washed twice with phosphate buffer saline (PBS), resuspended in PBS to a final concentration of 2×10^6 cells/ml, and used immediately for the experiments with the fluorescence activated cell sorter (FACS).

A single-cell fluorescence intensity analysis was quantitatively performed with the aid of a Becton-Dickinson FACS II. Excitation was performed with an argon laser at 288 nm, and fluorescence was detected at 530 nm. For calibration of the cell sorter, glutaraldehyde-fixed chick erythrocytes were used. For each measurement, a total of 4×10^4 cells were analyzed at a flow rate of 1000–1500 cells per second. The data obtained were displayed in the form of a histogram plotting cell number versus fluorescence intensity. The percentage of fluorescence was estimated from the number of fluorescent cells out of the 4×10^4 analyzed cells. In order to obtain further information regarding the distribution of fluorescence within a given population, the percentage of cells with low, intermediate, and high fluorescence was estimated by monitoring the percentage of fluorescent cells recovered in channels 513–660 (low fluorescence), 661–810 (intermediate fluorescence), and 811–1020 (high fluorescence). In all our measurements, the fluorescence background of unlabeled cells was less than 1%.

CONDITION FOR ACM EXPOSURE AND DETERMINATION OF INTRACELLULAR DRUG CONCENTRATION

Unless otherwise mentioned, 5×10^6 cells were exposed to drug in their respective fresh growth medium. For each drug concentration tested, at least two separate cultures were used.

After incubation with ACM, cells grown in suspension were washed in Hanks saline solution pH 7.2. ACM incorporated in total cells was extracted by resuspending the cell pellet in 1 ml Hanks solution containing 0.1% NP_{40}. After addition of 6 ml ethyl acetate, shaking and centrifugation at room temperature, the organic phase was evaporated, the dried pellet resuspended in the mobile phase, chloroform–methanol–acetic acid–water–triethylamine (68:20:10:2:0.01 v/v) and subjected to high pressure liquid chromatography (HPLC).

Results

INCORPORATION OF ADM, DNR, AND ACM INTO FLC

The uptake of ADM and DNR in FLC was analyzed by incubating 10^7 cells in a growth medium containing increasing amounts of ADM or DNR. Incubation was carried out at 37°C for 60 minutes. The cells were then washed twice with PBS, and fluorescence intensity at each concentration was analyzed with the cell sorter. As expected, the degree of fluorescence intensity was related to the drug concentration. When cells were incubated under the same conditions, a higher affinity was observed in the presence of DNR than in the presence of ADM (Table 1). This differ-

Table 1. Incorporation of Adriamycin and Daunorubicin in Friend Leukemia Cells at Different Concentrations[a]

Concentration of Drug (μg/ml)	Fluorescent Cells (%)		
	Low Intensity Range (513–660)	Inter-mediate Intensity Range (661–810)	High Intensity Range (811–1020)
1 ADM	100	0	0
1 DNR	98.9	11	0
3 ADM	100	0	0
3 DNR	75.2	24.1	0.7
10 ADM	91.7	8.0	0.3
10 DNR	63.7	18.1	18.2

[a]An amount of 10^7 FLC was incubated in 1 ml growth medium containing the appropriate concentration of ADM or DNR. Cells were incubated for 60 minutes at 37° C, washed twice with PBS, and the distribution of fluorescence was monitored with the aid of the FACS II as described in the text.

ential affinity could be related to a greater lipophilic character of DNR.

The kinetics of ACM uptake by sensitive FLC and its distribution observed in the cytoplasmic and the nuclear fractions were studied by incubating 5×10^6 cells in presence of 20 μg/ml ACM at 37°C. Uptake is a rapid process, more than 20% of the maximum uptake was in 5 seconds and found mainly in the nuclei. Maximum incorporation was obtained in 10–30 minutes and was followed by a decrease observed in nuclear fraction only. Although the mechanism of uptake is not known, it is assumed to be related to the dynamic structure of the cell membrane rather than to an active transport. This assumption was supported by the nonsignificant effect of the sodium azide. When cells were incubated at different temperatures, maximum uptake was observed at 37°C. At lower temperatures, however, uptake was reduced to be almost null at 0°C. Nuclear incorporation of ADM, DNR, and ACM did not appear to be affected by low temperatures, and uptake by isolated nuclei was about the same at 4°C and at 37°C.

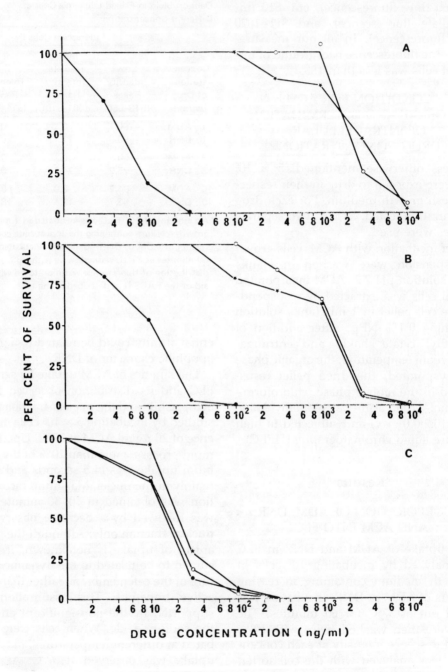

FIGURE 1. Cytotoxic effect of adriamycin, daunorubicin, and aclacinomycin A in FLC, ADM-RFLC, and DRN-RFLC. Friend leukemia cells (●) and the cell variants resistant to adriamycin (○) and to daunorubicin (⋆) were seeded at low density (0.1 × 10⁶/ml) in medium containing different amount of adriamycin (A), daunorubicin (B), or aclacinomycin (C). Cells were incubated 72 hours at 37 °C in a CO_2 incubator after which cells were counted using a hemacytometer and cell viability was measured by counting the cells excluding 0.1% trypan blue.

INCORPORATION OF ADM, DNR, AND ACM IN RESISTANT CELLS

Sublines of FLC resistant to ADM and to DNR were developed. The increase in resistance up to 100-fold was obtained, and cross-resistance was observed between ADM and DNR, but it was not observed with ACM (Fig. 1). The incorporation of ADM and DNR, correlated with size distribution, was analyzed on a single cell level with the aid of the FACS. From light-scattering measurements, the mean volume of ADM-RFLC was the same as that of sensitive cells. The fluorescence intensity of ADM-incorporated cells was related to the initial concentration but was lower in resistant cells. Changes in size distribution, characterized by an accumulation of small cells, was associated with resistance to DNR and not to ADM. Fluorescence distribution of DNR-incorporated cells revealed at least two populations of cells with different fluorescence intensity, mainly at a high initial concentration level. However, incorporation of these two drugs into isolated nuclei of resistant cells was not affected and was the same as in sensitive cells.

The kinetics of ACM uptake by ADM-RFLC and by DNR-RFLC, its rate of incorporation into the nuclei, and its intracellular metabolism was the same as in sensitive cells.

Our results suggest therefore that resistance to anthracycline is a consequence of changes induced in the plasma membrane components. Although cross-resistance between ADM and DNR was observed, the changes induced by these two drugs are probably due to different biochemical interactions. These changes did not interfere with the incorporation of aclacinomycin A.

Discussion

The anthracyclines were extensively investigated and little is known about the exact mode of cellular uptake.[11,23] In the present study, the incorporation of ADM, DNR, and ACM into FLC was monitored by the FACS II and HPLC, and fluorescence intensity was analyzed at the single cell level. Like others, we found a considerably slower uptake of ADM than DNR.[23,24] Since uptake of the three drugs is not inhibited by sodium azide, but it is time- and temperature-dependent, it is suggested that it occurs by a passive transport process across the cell membrane. The possibility that the composition and the dynamic structural organization of the cell surface membrane are associated with the rate of incorporation cannot be excluded. The nuclear incorporation, which is not hindered by sodium azide nor by low temperatures, is probably due to a different structural organization of the nuclear membrane. Cellular uptake is probably a decisive factor in the therapeutic effect of drugs belonging to this group. Therefore a decrease in cellular uptake can be an important cause of treatment failure.[25,26] The present study shows that resistance is due to a reduced uptake by the plasma membrane and not by the nuclear membrane. ADM-RFLC and DNR-RFLC are cross-resistant to ADM and to DNR but not to ACM.

We suggest therefore that the composition and the dynamic structural organization of the cell membrane are altered differently in ADM-RFLC and in DNR-RFLC. These changes did not affect the uptake of ACM.

ACKNOWLEDGMENTS

This work was supported by contract DGRST 80.7.0445 and by Simone and Cino Del Duca Foundation.

REFERENCES

1. Bernard J, Paul R, Boiron M, Jacquillat C, Maral R: *Rubidomycin: Recent Results in Cancer Research*. Springer-Verlag, Berlin, 1969.
2. Carter SK, Di Marco A, Ghione M, Krakoff IH, Mathé G (Eds): *International Symposium on Adriamycin, Milan 1971*. Springer-Verlag, Berlin, 1972.
3. Oki T, Matsuzawa Y, Yoshimoto A, Numata K, Kimatura I, Ori S, Takamatsu A, Umezawa H,

Ishizuka M, Naganawa H, Suda H, Hamada M, Takeuchi T: New antitumor antibiotics aclacinomycins A and B. *Jpn J Antibiot 28: 830–834, 1975.*

4. Skovsgaard T, Nissen NI: Adriamycin, an antitumor antibiotic: A review with special reference to daunomycin. *Dan Med Bull 22: 62–73, 1975.*

5. Whang-Peng J, Leventhal BG, Adamson JW, Petty S: The effect of daunomycin on human cells *in vivo* and *in vitro. Cancer 23: 113–121, 1969.*

6. Bachur NR, Hildebrand RC, Jaenke RS: Adriamycin and daunomycin disposition in the rabbit. *J Pharmacol Exp Ther 191: 331–340, 1974.*

7. Egorin MJ, Hildebrand RC, Cimino EF, Bachur NR: Cytofluorescence localization of adriamycin and daunorubicin. *Cancer Res 34: 2243–2245, 1974.*

8. Bachur NR: Anthracycline antibiotic pharmacology and metabolism. *Cancer Treat Rep 63: 817–820, 1979.*

9. Egorin MJ, Clawson RE, Ross LA, Schlossberger NM, Bachur N: Cellular accumulation and disposition of aclacinomycin A. *Cancer Res 39: 4396–4440, 1979.*

10. Atassi G, Tagnon HS, Bournonville F, Winands M: Comparison of adriamycin with DNA–adriamycin complex in chemotherapy of L1210 leukemia. *Eur J Cancer 10: 339–403, 1974.*

11. Meriwether WD, Bachur NR: Inhibition of DNA and RNA metabolism by daunorubicin and adriamycin in L1210 mouse leukemia. *Cancer Res 32: 1137–1142, 1972.*

12. Oki T: New anthracycline antibiotics. *Jpn J Antibiot Suppl. 30: 570–584, 1977.*

13. Pigram WJ, Fuller W, Hamilton LD: Stereochemistry of intercalation: Interaction of daunomycin with DNA. *Nature [New Biol] 235:17–19, 1972.*

14. Trouet A, De-Campeneere DD, De-Smedt-Malengreaux M, Atassi G: Experimental chemotherapy with a lysosmotropic adriamycin DNA complex. *Eur J Cancer 10: 405–411, 1974.*

15. Bhuyan BK, McGovren JP, Crampton SL: Intracellular uptake of 7-con-O-methylnogarol and adriamycin by cells in culture and its relationship to cell survival. *Cancer Res 41: 882–887, 1981.*

16. Krishan A, Israel M, Modest EJ, Frei E III: Differences in cellular uptake and cytofluorescence of adriamycin and N-trifluoroacetyl adriamycin-14-valerate. *Cancer Res 36: 2114–2116, 1976.*

17. Noel G, Peterson C, Trouet A, Tulkens P: Uptake and subcellular localization of daunorubicin and adriamycin in cultured fibroblasts. *Eur J Cancer 14: 363–368, 1978.*

18. Skovsgaard T: Transport and binding of daunorubicin, adriamycin and rubidazone in Ehrlich ascites tumor cells. *Biochem Pharmacol 26: 215–222, 1977.*

19. Yesair DW, Thayer PS, McNitt S, Teague K: Comparative uptake metabolism and retention of anthracyclines by tumors growing *in vitro* and *in vivo. Eur J Cancer 16: 901–907, 1980.*

20. Inaba M, Johnson RK: Uptake and retention of adriamycin and daunorubicin by sensitive and anthracycline resistant sublines of P388 leukemia. *Biochem Pharmacol 27: 2123–2130, 1978.*

21. Landos-Gagliardi D, Aubel-Sadron G, Maral R, Trouet A: Subcellular localization of daunorubicin in sensitive and resistant Ehrlich ascites tumor cells. *Eur J Cancer 16: 849–854, 1980.*

22. Seeber S, Loth H, Crooke ST: Comparative nuclear and cellular incorporation of daunorubicin, doxorubicin, carminomycin, marcellomycin, aclacinomycin A and AD 32 in daunorubicin sensitive and resistant Ehrlich ascites *in vitro. J Cancer Res Clin Oncol 98: 109–118, 1980.*

23. Noel G, Trouet A, Zenebergh A, Tulkens P: In *EORTC International Symposium Adriamycin Review* Staquet M, Tagnon H, Kenis Y, Bonadonna G, Carter SK, Sokal G, Trouet A, Ghione M, Praga C, Lenaz L, Karim OS (Eds), European Press: Medikon, Ghent, Belgium, 1975, p 99.

24. Tatsumi K, Nakamura T, Wakisaka G: Comparative effect of daunomycin and adriamycin on nucleic acid metabolism in leukemic cells *in vitro. Gan 65: 237–248, 1974.*

25. Chervinsky DS, Wang JJ: Uptake of adriamycin and daunorubicin in L1210 and human leukemia cells: A comparative study. *J Med 7: 63–79, 1976.*

26. Dano K: Active outward transport of daunomycin in resistant Ehrlich ascites tumor cells. *Biochim Biophys Acta 323: 466–483, 1973.*

CHAPTER 15

Covalent and Reversible Linkage of Daunorubicin to Proteins. Lysosomal Hydrolysis and Antitumoral Activity of Conjugates Prepared with Oligopeptidic Spacer Arms.

A. Trouet, R. Baurain, M. Masquelier, and D. Deprez-De Campeneere

The major technical problem in developing selective antitumor drug–protein conjugates is to obtain a covalent and reversible linkage between the drug and the carrier protein. This link should remain stable in the bloodstream and extracellular spaces and be sensitive to either the acidic pH or lysosomal enzymes to allow the *in situ* release of the drug under its active form after endocytosis of the conjugate.[1]

We have tackled this problem by linking the anthracycline drug daunorubicin (DNR) to bovine serum albumin (BSA) in such a covalent and reversible way. Using carbodiimide as a coupling agent, an amide bond was formed between the amino group of DNR, necessary for the activity of the drug, and the carboxylic side chains of the BSA.

Theoretically, such a peptidic linkage is unlikely to be split by peptidases due to steric hindrance and to the fact that such an amide bond is not adjacent to an asymmetric carbon.[2] However, by introducing an amino acid or an oligopeptidic

spacer arm between DNR and the carrier, we expected that the amide bond adjacent to DNR would become sensitive to peptidases, since this bond is now in the α position with regard to an asymmetric carbon. We expected also that by increasing the oligopeptidic chain length the steric hindrance would vanish and allow the enzymatic release of DNR from the conjugates.

To test our hypothesis, we synthesized various amino acid and peptidic derivatives of DNR by stepwise addition of the respective amino acids to the anthracyclines, as described previously.[3] They were then conjugated to serum albumin, using a soluble carbodiimide as condensing agent, and the conjugates were separated from the remaining free drugs by gel filtration on Bio-Gel P-100 and adsorption chromatography on Porapak Q.

The *in vitro* stability of the various BSA–anthracyclines conjugates in presence of serum or purified lysosomal peptidases has been determined by measuring the release of intact DNR using high pressure liquid chromatography and fluorometry.[4] In presence of 95% calf serum and at 37°C, less than 3% of DNR is released from the conjugate BSA–(a.a.)$_4$–DNR* after 24 hours of incubation. The influence of the peptidic spacer arm length on the release of DNR by a purified fraction of lysosomal

---

International Institute of Cellular and Molecular Pathology and Université Catholique de Louvain, Brussels, Belgium

*BSA–(a.a.)$_4$–DNR: Conjugate in which DNR is linked to BSA via four amino acids (a.a.).

101

enzymes[5] has been determined at pH 5.5. As illustrated in Figure 1, we confirmed experimentally that when DNR is linked directly to BSA ($n = 0$), no DNR can be liberated enzymatically from the BSA–DNR conjugate after 20 hours of incubation. As the length of the oligopeptidic spacer arm (1–4 amino acids) increases, the release of active DNR by the lysosomal enzymes increases. After 20 hours of incubation, 14, 30, and 44% of DNR are liberated from BSA–(a.a)$_1$–DNR, BSA–(a.a)$_2$–DNR, and BSA–(a.a)$_3$–DNR, respectively. More than 80% of DNR is released if a tetrapeptidic spacer arm is used to link DNR to the protein.

The therapeutic activity of the serum albumin–drugs conjugates has been studied in DBA/2 mice inoculated intraperitoneally with L1210 cells (Table 1). The conjugates were administered by the same route on days 1 and 2.

The carrier protein, BSA, as well as the conjugate formed by a direct linkage between DNR and this protein were completely devoid of activity. When the spacer arm is composed of one or two amino acids, the therapeutic activities are not greater than those observed with the optimal dose of DNR. On the other hand, when the oligopeptidic spacer arm consists in three or four amino acids, the con-

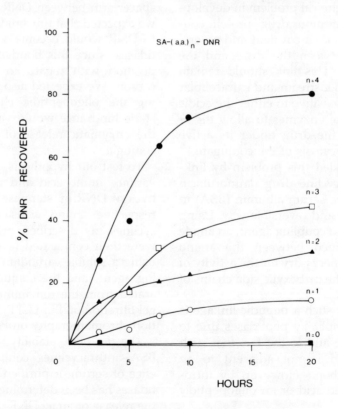

FIGURE 1. Influence of the length of the oligopeptidic spacer arm on the release, by lysosomal peptidases, of daunorubicin linked to serum albumin (SA). Daunorubicin linked to serum albumin (SA–(a.a)$_n$–DNR) directly ($n = 0$), via one amino acid ($n = 1$) or via a di-, tri-, or tetrapeptidic spacer ($n = 2$, 3, and 4, respectively) was incubated for up to 20 hours at 37°C and at pH 4.5 in presence of lysosomal enzymes purified from rat liver. The release of intact DNR was followed by high pressure liquid chromatography and fluorometry.

Table 1. Chemotherapeutic Activity of Serum Albumin-Daunorubicin Conjugates on Murine L1210 Leukemia[a]

Drug	Doses per Day (mg DNR/kg)	Doses per Day (mg BSA/kg)	Increase in Life Span (%)	No. of Survivors on Day 30/ Total No. of Mice	Weight Variation on Day 8 (%)
DNR	2	—	39	5/91	+0.4
	5	—	6	0/52	−12.3
BSA	—	59	−6	0/16	+9.1
	—	89	−1	0/8	+2.4
BSA-DNR	5	40	−2	0/7	+6.5
	5	51	9	0/9	+2.2
	7.5	77	8	0/10	+0.9
	7.5	77	9	0/6	−0.9
BSA-(a.a.)$_1$-DNR	5	49	6	0/10	+3.5
	7.5	74	6	0/10	−3.4
BSA-(a.a.)$_2$-DNR	5	41	30	0/10	−4.7
	7.5	62	33	0/10	−1.3
BSA-(a.a.)$_3$-DNR	5	29	>211	8/10	+0.4
	5	35	>200	6/10	+0.5
	7.5	43	>211	8/10	−7.9
	7.5	66	38	3/9	+2.1
	7.5	52	>200	7/10	−1.7
BSA-(a.a.)$_4$-DNR	5	39	107	4/10	−3.0
	5	58	26	0/8	+2.7
	5	40	>211	7/10	−3.9
	5	43	>189	5/9	+0.9
	7.5	59	>211	6/10	−9.8
	7.5	59	>211	10/10	−2.5
	7.5	59	>200	4/8	−4.4
	7.5	64	>189	7/9	−0.4

[a] 10^4 L1210 cells were inoculated I.P. on day 0 into DBA/2 mice. Drugs were given by the same route on days 1 and 2.

jugates are strikingly more active than DNR. Increases in life-span (ILS) greater than 200% are usually obtained. For the BSA-(a.a.)$_4$-DNR conjugate at 7.5 mg DNR equivalent/kg, more than 200% ILS and 73% long-term survivors are obtained.

In conclusion, we have developed a covalent and reversible linkage between an antitumor agent, DNR, and a protein that fulfills the criteria required for a lysosomotropic drug–carrier entity,[6] since the conjugate BSA-(a.a.)$_4$-DNR is stable in the bloodstream and releases in vitro the active DNR through the action of lysosomal enzymes. It could therefore be expected that in vivo this conjugate will be able to release DNR in the lysosomal compartment of the target cells after its endocytosis. We have

shown in the present study that a direct covalent linkage of DNR to BSA does not allow the lysosomal release of the active drug and leads to a conjugate that is completely devoid of antitumor activity in vivo against the I.P. inoculated L1210 murine leukemia. We have also observed that there is a correlation between the in vitro liberation of DNR by the lysosomal enzymes and the in vivo activity of the conjugates on the I.P. form of murine leukemia.

The covalent and reversible linkage we have developed could be used with other drugs and carriers. The drug bearing an amino group must be linked to its carrier protein through an oligopeptidic spacer arm composed of three or four amino acids, the nature and sequence of which should allow the release of the active drug by the lysosomal enzymes after endocytosis of the conjugate by the target cells. Serum albumin used in this study is not the ideal carrier for cancer chemotherapy. An ideal carrier must be recognized and endocytozed specifically by the cancer cells and will only be found by studying very carefully the receptors and the endocytosis of every cancer cell type.

REFERENCES

1. Trouet A, Deprez-De Campeneere E, de Duve C: Chemotherapy through lysosomes with a DNA–daunorubicin complex. *Nature [New Biol]* 239: 110–112, 1972.
2. Trouet A, Baurain R, Deprez-De Campeneere D, Layton D, Masquelier M: DNA, liposomes, and proteins as carriers for antitumoral drugs. *Recent Results Cancer Res* 75: 229–235, 1980.
3. Masquelier M, Baurain R, Trouet A: Amino acid and dipeptide derivatives of daunorubicin. 1. Synthesis, physicochemical properties and lysosomal digestion. *J Med Chem* 23: 1166–1170, 1980.
4. Baurain R, Deprez-De Campeneere D, Trouet A: Rapid determination of doxorubicin and its fluorescent metabolites by high-pressure liquid chromatography. *Anal Biochem* 94: 112–116, 1979.
5. Trouet A: Isolation of modified liver lysosomes. *Methods Enzymol* 31: 323–329, 1974.
6. Trouet A: Increased selectivity of drugs by linking to carriers. *Eur J Cancer* 14: 105–111, 1978.

CHAPTER 16

Daunomycin Targeting Using Carrier Monoclonal Antibodies

M. Page and J. P. Emond

Monoclonal antibodies were used for targeting daunomycin to the tumor cell. The drug was covalently bound to monoclonal antibodies directed against carcinoembryonic antigen (CEA) with 0.01% glutaraldehyde. The pharmacologic activity of the drug-antibody conjugate was assayed *in vitro* with human colon adenocarcinoma cells producing CEA. Using a drug to protein ratio of 5.7, the inhibition of thymidine incorporation was measured at various concentrations. AT 500 ng/ml, the activity of antibody-bound daunomycin was 800% the activity of an equivalent amount of free daunomycin; the activity of free antibody was only 2.2%, whereas the physical addition of both antibody and daunomycin gave 116% of the activity of the free drug alone. A 60-minute incubation period of the conjugate with adenocarcinoma cells was sufficient to obtain this effect. This new approach offers a potential application in cancer treatment, since the drug carrier is directed against an already used cancer marker.

Chemotherapeutic agents currently used for antitumor therapy are selected for their toxicity toward rapidly proliferating cells. Unfortunately, most of them cause undesirable systemic effects, such as cardiac or renal toxicity, bone marrow dysplasia, alopecia, and immunosuppression. During the last few years, many research-ers have tried to eliminate these side effects by increasing the availability of the drug for the tumor site. In this attempt, some have proposed to link these drugs with different kinds of macromolecules, such as proteins, enzymes or antibodies, lectins, toxins, or DNA.[1-8]

Antibodies against tumor-associated antigens have already been used mostly in animal models, but their use in human tumor treatment is limited, since no human tumor–specific surface antigen has been isolated and purified. The complexity of such a system would limit its clinical usefulness. However, human tumors often produce cancer-related oncofetal proteins that are being widely investigated and used as tumor markers in clinical monitoring.[9,10] Recently, Belles-Isles and Page[11,12] have reported two models of *in vitro* immunochemotherapeutic treatment of cancer cells with drug–antibody conjugates directed against two oncofetal proteins, alpha-fetoprotein and carcinoembryonic antigen (CEA).

We report the treatment *in vitro* of human colon adenocarcinoma cells (LoVo cells) producing CEA with daunomycin monoclonal anti-CEA conjugates.

Materials and Methods

LoVo cells, which produce CEA at a rate of 10 ng/day/10^6 cells, were kindly supplied by Dr. Ying Yang (M. D. Anderson Hospital, Houston, Texas). Daunomycin was purchased from Rhône-Poulenc, Paris,

Department of Biochemistry, Faculty of Medicine, Laval, University, Quebec, Canada

France; monoclonal antibody to CEA, from Hybritech, La Jolla, California; and glutaraldehyde from Sigma Chemicals, St. Louis, Missouri. RPMI 1640 culture medium (Flow Laboratories, Mississauga, Ontario, Canada) was supplemented with 10% fetal calf serum (Flow Laboratories).

PREPARATION OF DAUNOMYCIN—ANTI-CEA CONJUGATES

Daunomycin, 20 μg, and antibody, 100 μg, were dissolved in 75 μl of phosphate buffer saline at pH 7.2 and 10 μl of 0.1% glutaraldehyde in water were added. The solution was incubated for 10 minutes at 37°C. The free drug was separated from the conjugate by gel filtration on Sephadex G-50 (1 × 10 cm) equilibrated with 0.05 M ammonium acetate buffer at pH 6.5. The drug:protein ratio in the conjugate was evaluated by optical density at 495 nm for the drug and by the Lowry method for the protein content.[13] This procedure yielded a conjugate with a ratio of about 5 moles of drug per mole of protein.

INHIBITION OF THYMIDINE INCORPORATION

One million LoVo cells were incubated for 1 hour with free or bound daunomycin (0.1, 0.2, 0.5 μg/ml of culture medium) monoclonal anti-CEA or with a mixture of both substances; cells were then centrifuged at 4°C, washed in normal medium, and reincubated for another 2 hours with growth medium. A pulse of 1 μC of ^{3}H-thymidine (New England Nuclear, Montreal, Canada, 83 mC/mg), was added for 5 minutes at 37°C; 250 μl of cold 25% trichloroacetic acid was then added (final concentration, 5% W/V); the precipitated material was then centrifuged, washed three times, solubilized in 0.5 μl Protosol (New England Nuclear, Montreal, Canada), and counted in the presence of Scinti Verse (Fisher Scientific, Quebec, Canada). The radioactivity was counted in a RackBeta counter (LKB, Stockholm, Sweden).

Results

PHARMACOLOGIC ACTIVITY OF THE CONJUGATE

The inhibition of thymidine incorporation by LoVo cells after a short treatment with free or bound daunomycin (Fig. 1) shows that the conjugate retains both its immunologic and pharmacologic activity. At a drug concentration of 500 ng/ml, daunomycin monoclonal anti-CEA conjugate was eight times more active than the free drug. The physical addition of daunomycin and monoclonal antibody had some synergistic effect, but the total inhibition of thymidine incorporation was slightly better than the free drug. Free monoclonal anti-CEA causes a negligible inhibition of thymidine incorporation.

DOSE–RESPONSE RELATIONSHIP

The activity of daunomycin monoclonal anti-CEA was compared to that of the free

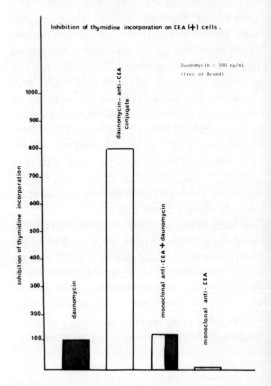

FIGURE 1. Inhibition of thymidine incorporation on CEA (+) producing cells (LoVo).

drug at 0.1, 0.2, and 0.5 μg/ml (Fig. 2). At each concentration, the inhibition of thymidine incorporation in the presence of the conjugates was at least twice that caused by the free drug at the same concentration. The conditions used for each assay were previously described.

Conclusion

We have already shown that antibodies directed toward oncofetal antigens present on the surface of tumor cells are efficient carriers of chemotherapeutic agents. Antimouse alpha-fetoprotein–daunomycin conjugates could inhibit growth and colony formation of mouse hepatoma cells.[11] We have reported recently that growth of human adenocarcinoma cells producing CEA was inhibited by treatment with daunomycin–anti-CEA conjugates.[12] The latter retains both their pharmacologic activity as demonstrated by inhibition of thymidine incorporation and their immunologic activity as determined by the lack of activity of the conjugates having no affinity for the target cell.

Preliminary data on the *in vivo* pharmacologic activity of daunomycin–anti-CEA conjugates, using LoVo cells grafted in nude mice, confirm these *in vitro* experiments. Non-specific side reactions are, however, expected, using the immunoglobulin fraction of monospecific antisera due to its polyclonal nature. The availability of monoclonal antibodies to human CEA offers a still better potential of application in cancer treatment, since it should eliminate most of the side effects encountered with monospecific antisera.

Our data show that the monoclonal conjugates retain both their pharmacologic and immunologic activity. One-hour treatment of LoVo cells with 500 ng/ml of conjugated daunomycin caused eight times more inhibition of thymidine incorporation than the free drug. This is the first application of monoclonal anti-CEA as a drug carrier for cancer treatment.

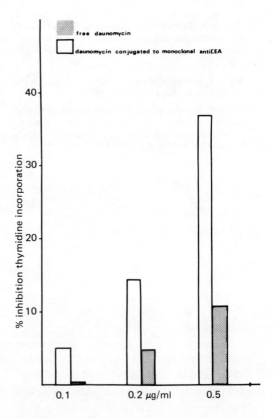

FIGURE 2. Relationship between the concentration of free or bound daunomycin and the inhibition of thymidine incorporation by LoVo cells.

REFERENCES

1. Lee FH, Berczy I, Fugimoto S, Sehon AH: The use of antifibrin antibodies for the destruction of tumor cells. *Cancer Immunol Immunother* 5: 201–206, 1978.
2. Ghose T, Norvell ST, Nigam SP: Antibody as carrier of chlorambucil. *Cancer* 29: 1398–1400, 1972.
3. Ghose T, Norvell ST, Guclu A, MacDonald AS: Immunochemotherapy of human malignant melanoma with chlorambucil carrying antibody. *Eur J Cancer* 11: 321–326, 1975.
4. Gregoriadis G: Targeting of drugs. *Nature* 265: 407–411, 1977.
5. Rowland GF, O'Neill GJ, Davies DAL: Suppression of tumor growth in mice by a drug–antibody conjugate using a novel approach to linkage. *Nature* 255: 487, 1975.
6. Mathé G, Baloc T, Bernard J: Effet sur la leucémie L-1210 de la souris d'une combinaison par diazotation d'Améthoptérine et de gamma-globulines de hamsters porteurs de cette leucémie par hétéro greffe. *CR Acad Sci (Paris)* 246: 1626, 1958.

7. Trouet A, Deprez-DeCampeneere D, DeDuve C: Chemotherapy through lysosomes with a DNA–daunorubicin complex. *Nature (New Biol)* 239: 110, 1972.

8. Kitao T, Hattori K: Concanavalin A as a carrier of daunomycin. *Nature* 265: 81, 1977.

9. Gold P, Freedman SO: Demonstration of tumor-specific antigens in human colonic carcinoma by immunological tolerance and absorption techniques. *J Exp Med 121: 439–443, 1965.*

10. Sell S, Becker FF: Alpha-fetoprotein. *J Natl Cancer Inst 60: 9–26, 1978.*

11. Belles-Isles M, Page M: *In vitro* activity of daunomycin–anti-alphafoetoprotein conjugates on mouse hepatoma cells. *Br J Cancer 41: 841, 1980.*

12. Belles-Isles M, Page M: Anti-oncofoetal proteins for targeting cytotoxic drugs. *Int J Immunopharmacol 3: 97–102, 1981.*

13. Lowry OH, Rosenbrough NJ, Farr AL, Randall RJ: Protein measurement with the Folin phenol reagent. *J Biol Chem 193: 265–269, 1951.*

CHAPTER 17

Effect of Temperature and Rate of Heating on Adriamycin-induced Cytotoxicity

T. S. Herman*

Introduction

Interest in hyperthermia as an anti-cancer treatment has been stimulated by laboratory studies that have shown enhanced cytotoxicity of several chemotherapeutic agents (including adriamycin) at elevated temperature. We have found, however, that the cytotoxicity caused by exposure to adriamycin at 42.4°C in Chinese hamster ovary (CHO) cells is decreased by about 0.5 log if heating to 42.4°C from 37°C is done over 3 hours (as is often required in patients undergoing whole body hyperthermia) rather than over <3 minutes as other *in vitro* investigations have utilized. In addition, in an attempt to develop a strategy that would result in an increased therapeutic index, we examined the effect of cooling as well as heating on the cytotoxicity of adriamycin. Cell killing by adriamycin was markedly inhibited by cooling during exposure, although prior cooling had no significant effect on the subsequent cytotoxic interaction between adriamycin and hyperthermia. The possible clinical relevance of these observations is that the entire body of patients being treated with adriamycin could be cooled using techniques now employed in cardiac surgery while large tumor masses could be heated using inductive heating methods now available. This approach might afford protection for the heart and bone marrow while maximizing antitumor effect.

The current burgeoning of interest in hyperthermia as an anticancer treatment stems from preclinical studies that have shown that cell killing associated with both selected antitumor drugs[8] and radiation[17] is greatly enhanced by hyperthermia. One of the first chemotherapeutic drugs to be studied systematically with hyperthermia was adriamycin. Hahn and Strande[9] showed that the cytotoxic interaction between adriamycin and hyperthermia was complex, being synergistic when cells were exposed to both agents briefly (≤30 minutes), but being antagonistic when the duration of combined exposure was longer or when exposure to hyperthermia substantially preceded treatment with adriamycin. We have also conducted laboratory investigations concerning the cytotoxic interaction between temperature alteration and adriamycin. We have been interested in adriamycin because of its wide spectrum of anticancer activity[3] and because synergistic cytotoxicity has been demonstrated for adriamycin and radiation[5] as well as for adriamycin and hyperthermia,[9] suggesting the possible utility of using all three modalities concurrently.

Department of Internal Medicine, Section of Hematology/Oncology, University of Arizona College of Medicine, Tucson, Arizona

*Present address: Department of Internal Medicine, Section of Hematology/Oncology, University of Arkansas, Little Rock, Arkansas.

Materials and Methods

METHOD OF CELL CULTURE

Chinese hamster ovary (CHO) cells were grown in McCoy's 5A medium supplemented with 20% (v/v) fetal calf serum, penicillin (11 units/ml), and strep-tomycin (100 μg/ml) (all from Grand Island Biological Co., Grand Island, New York). Cells were maintained in logarithmic growth phase at 37°C in a 5% CO_2–95% air atmosphere. Doubling time was 13–14 hours for the CHO cells. Cell numbers were determined with an electronic par-ticle counter (mode) ZBI, Coulter Elec-tronics, Hialeah, Florida).

CELL VIABILITY MEASUREMENTS

Cell viability was measured by the abil-ity of single cells to form colonies *in vitro*, as described previously.[6,7] The colony-forming efficiencies of control cultures was between 85 and 95%. The results from colony-forming experiments, described in graphs, represent at least three replicate experiments per figure.

TEMPERATURE AND DRUG TREATMENTS

Two sets of experiments will be report-ed. In the first set of experiments the effect of the rate of heating from 37–42.4°C on the cytotoxic interaction between adria-mycin and hyperthermia was determined. The temperature of 42.4°C was used be-cause we have found that it is the maxi-mum tolerable temperature for sustained (2–4 hours) whole-body hyperthermia treatments. In these investigations cells were heated from 37–42.4°C over times varying from ≤3 minutes to 3 hours (rates of heating between 1.8 and ≥108°C/hour). Cells were then maintained at 42.4°C and exposed to varying concentrations of adriamycin for 1 hour. Cell survival was determined by colony-forming ability, as already stated.

In the second set of experiments, the effect of cooling as well as heating cells during 1-hour exposures to adriamycin was determined. In these experiments, cells were cooled to 27, 30, or 32°C and ex-posed to varying concentrations of adria-mycin for 1 hour; or they were cooled to 30°C for 2 hours and then heated to 42.4°C over 30 minutes, and survival after exposure to varying concentrations of adriamycin for 1 hour was determined (drug was added after 42.4°C had been reached). Control cultures were exposed to varying concentrations of adriamycin for 1 hour at 37°C.

METHOD OF HEATING AND DRUG APPLICATIONS

Heating and cooling were accomplished in a plexiglass water tank with a con-tinuous in-flow and out-flow system con-nected to a Haake model FK water heater, as previously described.[10,11]

Small numbers of flasks were used so that all could be removed from the heating chamber, media poured off, and fresh media and drug added in less than 3 min-utes by a team of investigators. Drug solu-tions were always prepared immediately prior to use. After treatment, the medium was removed, and the cultures were washed twice with warmed Puck's saline A (Grand Island Biological Co.) and tryp-sinized (0.05% for 2–3 minutes). Follow-ing this, known numbers of cells were plated into plastic petri dishes for colony growth, as described above. Adriamycin was obtained from Farmetalia, Milan, Italy.

Results

Since our clinical studies with whole-body hyperthermia[13] indicated that the time required for raising core temperature to 42.4°C averaged 165 minutes when water circulation blankets were employed, we became interested in the effect on hyperthermic cell killing of the rate of heating to peak temperature. We had found and reported[15] that the rate of heating cells from 37–42.4°C determines the cytotoxicity observed at 42.4°C over time.

We next became interested in the effect of the rate of heating on cell killing due to chemotherapeutic drugs and hyperthermia. All previous *in vitro* studies[8] had utilized nearly immediately heating to test the cytotoxic interaction between various drugs and hyperthermia. Figure 1 shows the effect of the rate of heating on cytotoxicity due to exposure to 42.4°C and various concentrations of adriamycin for 1 hour. As can be seen, at concentrations above 0.2 mg/ml about 0.5 log less cell killing

occurs when heating from 37–42.4°C is conducted over 3 hours as opposed to immediately ($p < 0.1$ by the nonparametric Wilcoxin test[1]).

In the second set of experiments in this series we tested the effect on cell killing due to adriamycin of hypothermic as well as hyperthermic temperatures. In addition, we tested the effect of initial cooling on the cytotoxic interaction between adriamycin and hyperthermia. Figure 2 presents these data. When the temperature of exposure was varied from 27°C through 42.4°C, a family of survival curves was produced in which survival after 1-hour treatment with adriamycin was a function

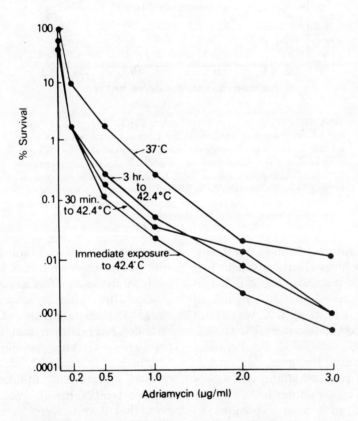

FIGURE 1. Effect of prior cooling on survival of CHO cells exposed to 42.4°C over the times indicated. CHO cells were cooled to 22°C for 2 hours and then heated to 42.4°C in 30 minutes and survival determined after maintenance at 42.4°C for the times indicated. Cells were also heated immediately to 42.4°C from 37°C (i.e., over ≤3 minutes) or were heated to 42.4°C from 37°C over 30 minutes and survival determined.

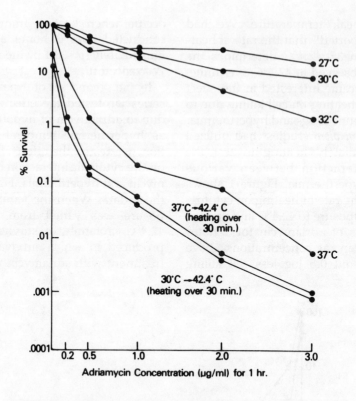

FIGURE 2.   Effect on survival of cooling CHO cells exposed to varying concentrations of adriamycin for 1 hour and the effect of prior
cooling on survival after exposure to adriamycin at 42.4°C. CHO cells
were cooled to the temperatures indicated and exposed to the concentration of adriamycin shown for 1 hour and survival determined.
Other CHO cells were cooled to 30°C for 2 hours and then heated over
30 minutes to 42.4°C, exposed to the concentrations of adriamycin
shown for 1 hour, and survival determined.

of the temperature during treatment.
Cooler temperatures clearly result in less
cell killing. For instance, the cell kill in
CHO cells exposed to 2.0 μg/ml of
adriamycin for 1 hour at 27°C was about
50%, as opposed to about 99.9% at 37°C
and about 99.99% at 42.4°C. Prior cooling
to 30°C for 2 hours, however, had no significant effect upon cell killing when cells
were heated over 30 minutes to 42.4°C and
then subjected to 1-hour exposures to
adriamycin.

Discussion

We have attempted to utilize our *in vitro*
cell system to suggest possibly useful clinical strategies for combining adriamycin
with temperature alteration. In our studies
we have made an effort to pattern investigations after clinically achievable parameters. The experiments of Hahn and
Strande[9] have shown that hyperthermia
produces striking synergism with
adriamycin (presumably because of increased adriamycin uptake at hyperthermic temperatures). We found, however, that if cells were heated to 42.4°C
over 3 hours (a time comparable with that
necessary to achieve a core temperature of
42.4°C in patients undergoing systemic
hyperthermia via heated water circulation
blankets[14]) then cell killing due to hyperthermia and adriamycin was decreased as

compared with the cytotoxicity achieved when faster rates of heating were employed. We also examined the effect upon adriamycin-induced lethality of hypothermic as well as hyperthermic temperatures and found that cell killing by adriamycin was a function of the temperatures during exposure (cooler temperatures protect).

A clinical trial of adriamycin and whole-body hyperthermia has been reported by Bull et al.[4] These investigators found that an adriamycin dose of 40 mg/m² was tolerable every 28 days with a core temperature of 41.8°C for 2 hours, although increased cardiotoxicity was a consequence.[15] Only 2 of 9 patients, however, achieved an objective response. Although the relative paucity of clinical activity was undoubtedly due to multiple factors, the fact that heating to peak temperatures required about 2 hours may have decreased the expected synergistic activity of the combination.

Using current knowledge, it may be possible to design better clinical trials utilizing adriamycin and temperature alteration. Since rapid heating results in maximum cytotoxic synergism between adriamycin and hyperthermia,[12] its use with regional-local hyperthermia may be most advantageous because heating times of 10–20 minutes are readily achievable using external devices now being perfected.[2] If the drug is to be used with whole-body hyperthermia, temperature elevation should probably be accomplished utilizing heating of extracorporally circulated blood as developed by Parks et al.[16] since this is the most efficient method to date and heating to 42.0°C can be accomplished in as little as 30 minutes.[17] It should be remembered, however, that rapid heating will also be more toxic to normal tissues, and maximum tolerable temperatures and drug doses may need to be redefined under these conditions.

In the future it may be possible to take full advantage of the interaction between the temperature of exposure and adriamycin cytotoxicity by inducing systemic hypothermia using extracorporeal circulation of blood (as is now done during cardiac surgery) and then to heat locally advanced tumors. Thus the heart and substantial portions of the bone marrow might be relatively spared adriamycin-induced toxicity, while antitumor effects should be maximized. Further, it is highly likely that temperature alteration and adriamycin will be combined with radiotherapy, but various aspects of this trimodality therapy will have to be carefully studied, since proper scheduling will depend on such factors as the microcirculation of tumors as well as direct cytotoxicity, and the understanding of these variables promises to be more complex than in the case of combining any two of these treatments.

ACKNOWLEDGMENTS

Supported in part by NIH Grant RO1 CA-26220 and Veterans Administration Research Support.

The author wishes to thank Eugene W. Gener for his continued assistance and support over years of collaboration.

REFERENCES

1. Armitage P: Wilcoxin's rank sum test. In *Statistical Methods in Medical Research*. New York, 1977, p 398.
2. Atkinson ER: Assessment of current hyperthermia technology. *Cancer Res* 39: 2313–2324, 1979.
3. Blum RH, Carter SK: Adriaymcin. A new anticancer drug with significant clinical activity. *Ann Intern Med* 80: 249–259, 1974.
4. Bull JM, Lees D, Schvette W, et al.: Whole body hyperthermia: A phase I trial of a potential adjuvant to chemotherapy. *Ann Intern Med* 90: 317–323, 1979.
5. Byfield JE, Lynch M, Kulhamian F, Chan PYM: Cellular effects of combined adriamycin and x-irradiation in human tumor cells. *Int J Cancer* 19: 194–204, 1977.
6. Gerner EW, Boone R, Connor WG, Hicks JA, et al.: A transient thermotolerant survival response produced by single thermal doses in HeLa cells. *Cancer Res* 36: 1035–1040, 1976.
7. Gerner EW, Schneider MJ: Induced thermal resistance in HeLa cells. *Nature* 256: 500–502, 1975.
8. Hahn GM: Potential for therapy of drugs and hyperthermia. *Cancer Res* 39: 2264–2268, 1979.

9. Hahn GM, Strande DP: Cytotoxic effects of hyperthermia and adriamycin on Chinese hamster cells. *J Natl Cancer Inst 57: 1063–1067, 1976.*

10. Herman TS, Cress AE, Sweets C, Gerner WS: Reversal of resistance to methotrexate by hyperthermia. *Cancer Res. (in press).*

11. *Herman TS, Gerner EW, Magun BE, et al.:* Rate of heating as a determinant of hyperthermia cytotoxicity. *Cancer Res.* In press.

12. Herman TS, Sweets CC, White DM, *et al.:* Effect of rate of heating on lethality due to hyperthermia and selected chemotherapeutic drugs. *J Natl Cancer Inst.* Submitted.

13. Herman TS, Zukoski CF, Anderson RM, *et al.:* Whole body hyperthermia and chemotherapy for treatment of patients with advanced, refractory malignancies. *Cancer Treat Rep.* In press.

14. Herman TS, Zukoski CF, Anderson RM: Whole body hyperthermia via water circulation techniques. *J Natl Cancer Inst.* In press.

15. Kim YD, Lees DE, Lake CR, *et al.:* Hyperthermia potentiates doxorubicin-related cardiotoxic effects. *JAMA 17: 1816–1817, 1979.*

16. Parks LC, Minaberry D, Smith DP, *et al.:* Treatment of far-advanced bronchogenic carcinoma by extracorporeally induced systemic hyperthermia. *J Thorac Cardiovasc Surg 78: 883–1979.*

17. Suit HD, Gerweck LE: Potential for hyperthermia and radiation therapy. *Cancer Res 39: 2290–2298, 1979.*

Part V

Clinical Studies
Classical Agents

CHAPTER 18

Pharmacokinetics of Adriamycin

J. Robert and B. Hoerni

Studying what happens to a drug in an organism may allow important practical benefits in its clinical use.

A good knowledge of the pharmacokinetics of a drug may considerably increase its clinical use: selection of the 1) administration route, 2) schedule of repetitive administrations (which is especially important in oncology), 3) coupling molecules, 4) new therapeutic agents inside a group of related structures, and 5) associated therapies that might increase the availability of the drug to its sites of action.

The pharmacokinetic study of a drug appears as the connection of three requirements: 1) a good analytical method, precise and sensitive enough to allow serial routine determinations; 2) a good mathematical processing of the analytical data, allowing a possible modelization; 3) the availability of homogeneous groups of cancer patients receiving well-defined chemotherapy regimen.

The pharmacokinetics of adriamycin in cancer patients has been studied in some detail by several authors.[1-8] We report here on recent findings we obtained in locally advanced breast cancers and non-Hodgkin's lymphomas.

Experimental

THE ANALYTICAL PROBLEM

We are using the technique presented by Israël et al.[9] with minor modifications.

Separation is achieved with a Waters Associates chromatograph, on a microbondapak-phenyl column (30 × 0.4 cm) with an isocratic solvent mixture (0.1% ammonium formate buffer pH 4.0/acetonitrile, 32/68, v/v). The solvent flow is 3 ml/min. The peaks are detected on a Schoeffel model SF 970 fluorometer with an excitation wavelength of 254 nm and an emission cut off filter at 580 nm. Recording and integration of the peaks allow the quantification of the fluorescence detection, using daunorubicin as an internal standard.

We have developed an original extraction technique that tentatively avoids the drawbacks of the classic extraction techniques. We are using minichromatographic open columns (Sep-pak, Waters Associates) as already described.[10] Solvents or fluids are pushed through the column with a glass syringe. Equilibration of the cartridge is obtained by running successively: 1) 3 ml methanol, 2) 3 ml methanol/water 1/1 (v/v); 3) 10 ml buffered sodium phosphate 0.05 M, pH 7.0. The plasma or urine sample (0.2–3 ml) is then pushed through the Sep-pak; washing with buffered sodium phosphate eliminates most of the constituents of serum from the Sep-pak. Elution of anthracyclines is then obtained with chloroform/methanol 1/1 (v/v) or pure methanol. This eluate, after evaporation and reconstitution in a small volume of the high pressure liquid chromatography (HPLC) mobile phase, can be injected in the chromatograph. We have demonstrated that this technique leads to almost quantitative recoveries of all the anthracyclines and metabolites tested; re-

Fondation Bergonié, Bordeaux, France

covery is linear up to very high concentrations of drug (5000 ng/ml).

THE MATHEMATICAL PROBLEM

The mathematical analysis of the data must be performed at different successive levels: 1) calculation of the equation of the plasma decay curves obtained for the parent drug and its metabolites; 2) modelization of the results in order to propose a type of distribution of the drug in the organism. The first point leads to macroconstants, which can be obtained using a computer program based upon successive linear regressions or upon nonlinear fittings. The second point leads to microconstants describing the behavior of the drug in the organism; it needs the knowledge of the elimination routes and metabolites and requires several assumptions that may not be easily demonstrable.

The analysis of the plasma decay curve of adriamycin after an I.V. bolus shows the existence of three successive phases. This three-phase kinetics was also observed by several authors,[2,3] whereas others postulated rather a two-phase kinetic behavior.[1,6] Calculation of the macroconstants is based upon Equation 1.

$$C_t = Ae^{-\alpha t} + Be^{-\beta t} + Ce^{-\gamma t} \qquad (1)$$

in which C_t is the plasma concentration at any time; A, B, and C are the intercepts of the three exponential lines with the Y axis; α, β, and γ are the slopes of these three straight lines, the sum of which is the curve observed.

These macroconstants A, B, C, α, β, and γ allow the determination of the total plasmatic clearance of the drug:

$$Cl = \frac{q}{AuC} \qquad (2)$$

in which q is the dose injected and AuC is the area under the curve, which is given by Equation 3:

$$AuC = \frac{A}{\alpha} + \frac{B}{\beta} + \frac{C}{\gamma} \qquad (3)$$

The macroconstants α, β, and γ also allow the calculation of the three successive half-lives of the drug in plasma (Equation 4):

$$t_{1/2} = \frac{Ln2}{\alpha}, \frac{Ln2}{\beta}, \frac{Ln2}{\gamma} \qquad (4)$$

THE CLINICAL PROBLEM

In order to obtain useful data from pharmacokinetic studies, it is necessary to obtain homogenous groups of patients behaving similarly from a clinical point of view. It is then possible to study the variability of the kinetic parameters and to compare it to the variability of the clinical responses. The first group of patients had locally advanced breast tumor that could not be surgically removed. A reliable measurement of the tumor mass can be obtained at various stages of the treatment and can be used as an indication of therapeutic efficacy.

These patients received combination chemotherapy consisting of adriamycin (50 mg/m^2) on day 1, vincristine (1 mg/m^2) on day 2, and methotrexate (6 mg/m^2) on days 3, 4, and 5. Adriamycin was injected as an I.V. bolus for about 3 minutes. In this protocol five similar courses were performed at 3 week intervals[11] before any local specific treatment. It must be kept in mind that there were several limitations to this study: 1) the entry of patients in the experimental protocol was low for different reasons, the main one being the peripheral vein status; 2) although pharmacokinetics was evaluated after the injection of adriamycin alone, the clinical response was evaluated after the injection of the whole chemotherapy; 3) it was impossible, for ethical considerations, to measure the pharmacokinetic parameters and the clinical response for every chemotherapy course of every patient. The first course was the only one to be studied in most cases.

In a second study we determined the pharmacokinetics of adriamycin in a group of patients with non-Hodgkin's lymphomas, who had received several injections of adriamycin on various schedules of administration. This allowed us to get some information about the time- and dose-dependence of the kinetics of this drug. Some of the determinations were performed only on the very early phase of the pharmacokinetics, during the first 30 minutes after administration. Such measurements allowed the determination of only the α phase of the kinetics. The "early clearance" was determined using Equation 5:

$$Cl = \frac{dose}{\frac{A}{\alpha}} \quad (5)$$

Comparison between the early phase kinetics and the whole pharmacokinetics in several patients has demonstrated the identity of the α phase in both types of determination. Moreover, the early clearance is fairly well correlated with the total plasmatic clearance. These early phase studies can therefore be considered as representative of the complete study.

Results and Discussion

In the first group of patients (locally advanced breast cancer) a comparison between pharmacokinetics parameters and short-term clinical response has been made. The α, β, and γ parameters presented small individual variations, and the half-lives were 4.72 $\pm$1.5 minutes, 1.26 $\pm$0.6 and 21.3 $\pm$7.4 hours. No correlation was observed between these values and the clinical response. Parameters A, B, and C, on the opposite, were much more scattered and individual values ranged between 1,939 and 15,800 ng/ml for A, between 22 and 245 ng/ml for B, and from 20 to 74 ng/ml for C.

Moreover, a significative correlation exists between the short-term clinical response and the A and B parameters (Fig. 1), this correlation being particularly significant for the early phase. No correlation, however, did exist between the long-term clinical response and any of the pharmacokinetic parameters.

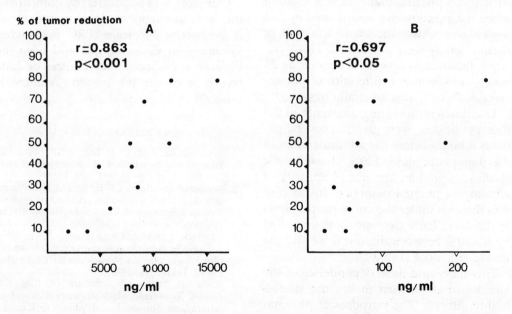

FIGURE 1.   Clinical response versus A and B parameters.

The existence of a correlation between a clinical response and the pharmacokinetic parameters of a drug must be emphasized. The existence of such a correlation makes it necessary to develop further work on the individual adaptation of therapeutic doses in function of the pharmacokinetic parameters measured in individual patients.

From the results obtained in the second group of patients (non-Hodgkin's lymphomas), we can assume the time- and dose-dependence of adriamycin pharmacokinetics. We had already observed by single-point measurements[12] that a decrease of adriamycin plasma levels occurred between the first injection and the following ones. Considering the whole phamacokinetics, successive injections in a patient with the same dosage did not provide similar pharmacokinetic parameters. The α, β and γ coefficients were not significantly altered, but the A, B, and C parameters were highly modified, especially parameter A. The area under the curve was generally reduced by 20–60% at the second injection; in one patient, however, this value was increased in the same proportion. This time-dependence of adriamycin pharmacokinetics was evident when the injections were separated by 2–3 weeks when two successive courses of chemotherapy were performed. However, when the injections were separated by 24 hours, no significant difference of parameters A, B, or C was generally observed.

Test doses representing one-tenth of the therapeutic dose were given in several patients 6 hours before the administration of the therapeutic dose. Early phase kinetic studies showed an absence of linearity of adriamycin pharmacokinetics. In no case was the area under the curve proportional to the dose. Early clearance was increased by 40–70% between the test dose and the therapeutic dose (Table 1).

This time- and dose-dependence of the kinetics of adriamycin makes the studies highly difficult. The purposes of pharmacokinetic studies are 1) individual adaptation of doses; 2) proposition of new therapeutic schedules; with a time- and dose-dependent model, the individual adaptations of therapeutic doses become much more complicated. It is evident that it is important to perform these studies in order to be able to give similar drug exposures to similar patients.

Table 1. Time- and Dose-Dependence of Adriamycin Pharmacokinetics[a]

	Test Dose (1/11)	Therapeutic Dose (10/11)	Difference (%)
Patient 1	1251 ml·min^{-1}	1750 ml·min^{-1}	+40
Patient 2			
First	1180	2097	+72
Second	1542	2893	+88
Difference	+31%	+43%	
Patient 3			
First	1332	2210	+66
Second	2186	3094	+42
Difference	+64%	+40%	

[a]Values of the "early clearances" in three patients according to the dose and to the number of courses.

ACKNOWLEDGMENTS

Our work was supported by grants from the Institut National de la Santé et de la Recherche Médicale (PRC Recherches Cliniques en Cancérologie) and from the Fédération Nationale des Centres de lutte contre le cancer (Opération "Vaincre le cancer").

REFERENCES

1. Benjamin RS, Riggs CE Jr, Bachur NR: Pharmacokinetics and metabolism of adriamycin in man. *Clin Pharmacol Ther* 14: 592–600, 1973.
2. Benjamin RS, Riggs CE Jr, Bachur NR: Plasma pharmacokinetics of adriamycin and its metabolites in humans with normal hepatic and renal function. *Cancer Res* : 1416–1420, 1977.
3. Chan KK, Cohen JL, Gross JF, *et al.*: Prediction of adriamycin disposition in cancer patients using a physiologic, pharmacokinetic model. *Cancer Treat Rep* 62: 1161–1171, 1978.
4. Reich SD, Steinberg G, Bachur NR, Riggs CE, Goebel R, Berman M: Mathematical model for adriamycin (doxorubicin) pharmacokinetics. *Cancer Chemother Pharmacol* 3: 125–131, 1979.

5. Chan KK, Chlebowski RT, Tong M, Chen HSG, Gross JF, Bateman JR: Clinical pharmacokinetics of adriamycin in hepatoma patients with cirrhosis. *Cancer Res 40: 1263–1268, 1980*.

6. Ehninger G, Stocker HJ, Proksch B, Wilms K: Die Pharmacokinetik von Adriamycin und Adriamycin-Metaboliten. *Klin Wochenschr 58: 927–934, 1980*.

7. Lee YTN, Chan KK, Harris PA, Cohen JL: Distribution of adriamycin in cancer patients. Tissue uptakes, plasma concentration after IV and hepatic IA adminstration. *Cancer 45: 2231–2239, 1980*.

8. Piazza E, Donelli MG, Broggini M, *et al.*: Early phase pharmacokinetics of doxorubicin (adriamycin) in plasma of cancer patients during single or multiple-drug therapy. *Cancer Treat Rep 64: 845–854, 1980*.

9. Israël M, Pegg WJ, Wilkinson PM, Garnick MB: Liquid chromatographic analysis of adriamycin and metabolites in biological fluids. *J Liq Chromatogr 1: 795–809, 1978*.

10. Robert J: Extraction of anthracyclines from biological fluids for HPLC evaluation. *J Liq Chromatogr 3: 1561–1572, 1980*.

11. Chauvergne J, Durand M, Hoerni B, Cohen P, Lagarde C: La chimiothérapie d'induction dans les cancers du sein à haut risque. Résultats d'une étude thérapeutique prospective. *Bull Cancer (Paris) 66: 9–16, 1979*.

12. Gessner T, Robert J, Bolanowska W, *et al.*: Effects of prior therapy on plasma levels of adriamycin during subsequent therapy. *J Med. 12: 183–193, 1981*.

CHAPTER 19

Adjuvant Doxorubicin Therapy of Solid Tumors

R. J. Brooks

With improved understanding of tumor biology, it is now apparent that many cancers are disseminated at the time of initial presentation. Local treatment modalities, such as surgery or radiotherapy, may well be successful in controlling a primary tumor only to be followed by the development of gross metastatic disease arising from previously unrecognized micrometastases. For this reason, interest has emerged in the addition of systemic adjuncts to the local treatment of malignancy. This approach has primarily involved the use of cytotoxic drugs, administered with the intent of eliminating micrometastatic deposits. Particular success has been met in the management of breast cancer. Many reports are now available detailing the effects of adjuvant chemotherapy, usually applied to the treatment of patients with regionally metastatic breast cancer.[1-3] This report will focus largely on the results of adjuvant breast cancer treatment programs utilizing the anthracycline doxorubicin (adriamycin). Brief mention will also be made of an anthracycline-based adjuvant treatment program for osteosarcoma.

The Arizona Adjuvant Breast Cancer Trials

Adjuvant trials for breast cancer at the University of Arizona began in 1974. Our regimen utilized a combination of adria-

University of Arizona, Cancer Center, Tucson, Arizona

mycin and cyclophosphamide (AC). This combination was selected because of demonstrated activity in the treatment of advanced breast cancer, ease of administration, and relative lack of toxicity.[4] Evidence was also available suggesting drug synergism.[5] Our initial trial for Stage II breast cancer was modified in 1975 by the addition, on a randomized basis, of regional radiotherapy. That same year a pilot trial for node-negative carcinoma of the breast was also begun.

Methods

Following surgery, patients with primary breast cancer ≤5 cm in diameter, with or without axillary lymph node involvement (Stage I or II), were referred for possible inclusion in this trial. Patients were carefully evaluated for the presence of metastatic disease. A thorough physical examination with routine screening laboratory tests and a radionuclide bone scan were obtained on all patients. Appropriate radiographs were obtained if abnormalities were present on bone scan. Unless obvious destructive changes were identified on x-rays, or other evidence of metastases discovered, the patient was considered eligible. Pathologic review was requested on all patients. Patients with bilateral or prior breast cancer or heart disease were excluded.

Adjuvant AC chemotherapy was initiated within 2 months of surgery. Adriamycin was administered at 30 mg/m² intravenously on day 1, and cyclophosphamide was given orally at 150 mg/m² on days 3 through 6 of each treatment cycle. This cycle was repeated at 3-week intervals. Patients with T1N0 lesions received three courses of AC for a total adriamycin dose of 90 mg/m². During the initial phase of this trial, patients with T2N0 lesions received three courses of AC as well. Following an early T2N0 relapse, however, the study design was changed so that these patients would receive eight courses of AC, resulting in a total adriamycin dose of 240 mg/m². Postoperative radiotherapy, although not part of the study design for node-negative patients, was permissible. Patients with Stage II (T1 or T2, N1) breast cancer were randomized to receive eight cycles of AC chemotherapy with or without regional radiotherapy. Radiotherapy (4400 rads) was administered following the second course of AC and was followed by six more cycles of AC.

Once patients completed their prescribed course of adjuvant treatment, they were followed off all therapy and reexamined every 3 months. A complete blood count and liver function tests were obtained at each visit. A chest radiograph was obtained every 6 months. Radionuclide bone scanning and mammography of the remaining breast were performed yearly. Histologic confirmation of relapse was made whenever feasible. Relapse-free and overall survival were calculated by the method of Kaplan and Meier.[6]

Results

Since 1975, 80 eligible node-negative patients have been entered in this study. Thirty-four patients had T1N0 lesions and 46 patients had T2N0 lesions. Patients ranged in age from 26 to 73 years. Seventy-five percent of the patients were between the ages of 40 and 69 years. Tumors occurred most commonly in the lateral portion of the breast (55%), although 22% occurred medially. Menopausal status was assessed for each patient. Twenty-nine patients (36%) were premenopausal and 51 patients (64%) were postmenopausal.

Fifty-eight patients (73%) received a modified radical mastectomy, with 20 patients undergoing radical mastectomy and 2 patients in this series receiving lumpectomy. Although routinely obtained at the present time, estrogen receptor (ER) determination was performed infrequently when this study was initiated; data on ER are available for 22 patients. The mean number of axillary lymph nodes removed was 15 in both the T1N0 and T2N0 groups.

Twenty-nine patients with T1N0 lesions received three courses of AC. Five T1N0 patients received eight courses. These patients had been initially classified as having T2N0 lesions but upon further pathologic review, were reassigned to the T1N0 group. Patients with T2N0 lesions were almost evenly divided between those receiving three courses (25 patients, 54%) and eight courses (21 patients, 46%) of AC. Bonnadonna's group[7] has recently reported on the importance of cytotoxic drug dosage in the adjuvant treatment of breast cancer. Of note, 60 patients, or 75% of the entire group, received greater than 85% of the calculated protocol dose of AC. A treatment delay, often the result of postoperative radiotherapy, occurred in 11 patients. Ten patients, three in the T1N0 group and seven in the T2N0 group, received postoperative radiotherapy.

To date, there have been two relapses among 80 node-negative patients treated with adjuvant AC. Median follow-up for the entire group is 40 months. Thus far, there have been no relapses among 34 patients in the T1N0 group. Two relapses have occurred in the T2N0 group. Both of these patients were premenopausal. One patient received three cycles of AC and relapsed 10 months following the completion of treatment. The second patient received eight courses of AC plus adjuvant radiotherapy and relapsed 25 months following the last course of chemotherapy. Thus, at the present time, 78 of 80 patients remain disease-free. Relapse-free survival (RFS) for the entire group of node-negative patients has been compared to a computer-based historical control group (the "Natural History Data Base") and the difference is statistically significant ($p <$ 0.01).[8]

Since 1974, 159 eligible patients with Stage II breast cancer were entered in this study and considered evaluable. Ninety-six patients received AC and 63 patients received AC plus radiotherapy (AC/XRT). There was a slight imbalance in age distribution with more older patients in the AC group as compared to the group receiving AC/XRT. Patients were otherwise similar in both treatment groups according to tumor size, tumor location, and menopausal status. Most patients (69%) were postmenopausal. ER status was known in 43 patients. Twenty-four patients receiving AC/XRT and 63 patients receiving AC alone had one to three positive nodes. Thirty-six patients in the AC/XRT group and 33 patients in the AC group had more than three positive nodes. Again, the majority of patients (78%) received greater than 85% of the calculated protocol dose of AC.

No statistical difference in RFS was noted between premenopausal and post-menopausal patients ($p = 0.15$). RFS in patients with greater than three positive nodes was significantly poorer than in those patients with one to three nodes ($p < 0.001$). Overall, there was no significant difference in RFS between the two treatment groups (AC vs AC/XRT, $p = 0.92$). However, when nodal status was considered, an interesting observation was made. Patients with one to three positive nodes had improved RFS when treated with AC/XRT as compared to those who received AC alone ($p = 0.05$). This difference was not observed in patients with greater than three positive nodes ($p = 0.95$).

We next analyzed type of relapse (loco-regional vs systemic) for all cases by treatment and nodal status. For the group as a whole, no difference was observed in the number of locoregional or distant recurrences between the two treatment groups. When broken down into subgroups by nodal status and treatment, however, a difference was suggested. In patients with one to three positive nodes, there were more locoregional relapses in patients who received AC alone. This difference was not seen in patients with more than three positive nodes.

Toxicity was minimal. Alopecia was common, but markedly reduced in those patients receiving scalp hypothermia during adriamycin infusion.[9] Some patients experienced mild nausea and vomiting. Significant leukopenia or thrombocytopenia was uncommon. Serious bacterial infection occurred in less than 1% of the patients. No long-term sequelae, such as second malignancies or leukemia, have been observed. No patient has manifested adriamycin cardiotoxicity.

Other Adriamycin-Based Adjuvant Breast Treatment Programs

Another major anthracycline-based adjuvant breast cancer trial has been conducted (during the same time period as the Arizona trial) by the M. D. Anderson group. A recent update of this study was presented at the Third International Conference on the Adjuvant Therapy of Cancer held in March 1981 in Tucson, Arizona.[10] The M. D. Anderson regimen utilized a combination of 5-fluorouracil (5-FU), adriamycin, and cyclophosphamide (FAC) plus BCG immunotherapy. Since 1974, 222 patients with Stage II and III breast cancer have been treated with this program. When compared with historical controls, statistically significant improvement in RFS was observed in both the Stage II and Stage III groups. Similarly, survival for the entire group was significantly better than that of the control group ($p < 0.01$).

Conclusion

Combined results of the University of Arizona and M. D. Anderson trials indicate the efficacy of anthracycline-based chemotherapy regimens in the treatment of all stages (I, II, III) of early breast cancer. These results are not surprising in view of the high degree of activity of single-agent adriamycin in the treatment of advanced breast cancer.[11] These data would indicate that anthracyclines should continue to play a key role in the planning of future adjuvant treatment protocols for breast cancer, although long-term analysis of toxicity (e.g., late cardiotoxicity) will be crucial in assessing the role of anthracycline-based treatment compared to other regimens (e.g., cyclophosphamide, methotrexate, 5-FU).

Adjuvant Treatment of Osteosarcoma

Five-year survival for osteosarcoma following surgery and/or radiotherapy is approximately 20%, with most patients eventually succumbing to widely disseminated disease.[12] Several reports have appeared documenting the efficacy of adriamycin in the adjuvant treatment of osteosarcoma.[13,14]

High-dose methotrexate (HDMTX) followed by citrovorum factor rescue has also been reported to improve RFS following primary treatment.[15] The Cancer and Leukemia Group B has recently reported an updated comparison of adjuvant treatment with adriamycin alone versus adriamycin alternating with HDMT.[16] In this trial, 99 patients were randomized to receive either adriamycin, 30 mg/m² I.V. daily for 3 consecutive days every 4 weeks for six courses, or adriamycin, two courses, alternating with two courses of HDMTX with citrovorum factor. Adriamycin and HDMTX were alternated for a total of six courses of each drug. Criteria for entry included histologic verification of diagnosis, complete resection without evi-

dence of residual disease, adequate bone marrow function, normal renal function, absence of obvious heart disease, and the requirement that no prior chemotherapy or radiotherapy had been given. Patients with parosteal sarcoma, chondrosarcoma, fibrosarcoma, radiation-induced osteosarcoma, soft tissue sarcoma, and osteosarcoma associated with Paget's disease were excluded.

Eighty-nine of the 99 patients were evaluable. Fifty-one were randomized to receive adriamycin alone and 38 to receive combination treatment with adriamycin and HDMTX. Patients were well matched with respect to sex, age, and tumor size. More tibial primaries occurred in the combined treatment group, but both groups were otherwise well matched with respect to site of primary tumor.

Regardless of tumor size, RFS was superior in the group receiving adriamycin alone. The advantage of single-agent adriamycin was seen in females but not in males and in patients over but not under the age of 16 years. Among patients with primary lesions in the femur, RFS was superior among patients receiving adriamycin alone ($p = 0.04$). Life table analysis estimates at 36 months indicate 82% of the patients in the adriamycin group to be alive vs 57% in the adriamycin/ HDMTX group ($p = 0.03$). An interesting finding was that, even following relapse, survival was superior in the group receiving adriamycin alone. Since the total dose of adriamycin is identical in both groups, drug scheduling may be extremely important.

Summary

An attempt has been made to review two major areas in which adjuvant treatment regimens utilizing the anthracycline adriamycin appear to have impacted significantly upon the natural history of malignant disease. With improved understanding of the biochemistry and pharmacology of presently available anthracyclines, the development of new agents, and the possibility of modifying adriamycin cardiotoxicity, the anthracycline class of anticancer drugs should continue to play an ever-increasing role in the adjuvant treatment of cancer.

REFERENCES

1. Bonadonna G, Brusamolino E, Valagussa P, et al.: Combination chemotherapy as an adjuvant treatment in operable breast cancer. N Engl J Med 294: 405–410, 1976.
2. Rivkin S, Glocksberg H, Rasmussen S: Adjuvant chemotherapy in Stage II breast cancer. In Adjuvant Therapy of Cancer III, Salmon S, Jones S (Eds). Grune & Stratton, New York, 1981.
3. All participating NSABP Investigators, Fisher B: Breast cancer studies of NSABP. In Adjuvant Therapy of Cancer III, Salmon S, Jones S (Eds). Grune & Stratton, New York, 1981.
4. Jones S, Durie B, Salmon S: Combination chemotherapy with adriamycin and cyclophosphamide for advanced breast cancer. Cancer 36: 90–97, 1975.
5. Corbett TH, Griswold DP, Mayo JG, et al.: Cyclophosphamide-adriamycin combination chemotherapy of transplantable murine tumors. Cancer Res 35: 1568–1573, 1975.
6. Kaplan E, Meier P: Non-parametric estimations from incomplete observations. J Am Stat Assoc 53: 457–481, 1958.
7. Bonadonna G, Valagussa P: Dose response effect of adjuvant chemotherapy in breast cancer. N Engl J Med 304: 10–15, 1981.
8. Moon TE, Jones SE, Davis SL, et al.: Development of a natural history data base for breast cancer. In Adjuvant Therapy of Cancer III, Salmon S, Jones S (Eds). Grune & Stratton, New York, 1981.
9. Dean JD, Salmon SE, Griffith KS: Prevention of doxorubicin-induced hair loss with scalp hypothermia. N Engl J Med 301: 1427–1429, 1979.
10. Buzdar A, Smith T, Blumenschein G, et al.: Adjuvant chemotherapy with fluorouracil, doxorubicin and cyclophosphamide (FAC) for stage II or III breast cancer: Five-year results. In Adjuvant Therapy of Cancer III, Salmon S, Jones S (Eds). Grune & Stratton, New York, 1981.
11. Hoogstraten B, George SC, Samal B: Combination chemotherapy and adriamycin in patients with advanced breast cancer. Cancer 38: 13–20, 1976.
12. Friedman MA, Carter SK: The therapy of osteogenic sarcoma: Current status and thoughts for the future. J Surg Oncol 4: 482–510, 1972.
13. Cortes EP, Holland JF, Glidewell O: Amputation and adriamycin in primary osteosarcoma: A five-year report. Cancer Treat Rep 62: 271–277, 1978.
14. Fossati-Bellani F, Gasparini M, Gennari L, et al.: Adjuvant treatment with adriamycin in primary operable osteosarcoma. Cancer Treat Rep 62: 279–281, 1978.
15. Rosenberg SA, Chabner BA, Young RC, et al.: Treatment of osteogenic sarcoma: Effect of adjuvant high dose methotrexate after amputation. Cancer Treat Rep 63: 739–751, 1979.
16. Cortes EP, Necheles T, Holland JF, et al.: Adjuvant chemotherapy for primary osteosarcoma: A cancer and leukemia group B experience. In Adjuvant Therapy of Cancer III, Salmon S, Jones S (Eds). Grune & Stratton, New York, 1981.

CHAPTER 20

Combination Chemotherapy with Adriamycin and BCG Immunotherapy as an Adjuvant Treatment of Breast Cancer: Preliminary Results of Two Randomized Trials

Group Inter France*

The long-lasting increase of disease-free survival obtained by adjuvant combination chemotherapy is now fairly well established for localized breast cancer in premenopausal women.[1-3] In postmenopausal patients some trials indicate better results from combination chemotherapy with more intensive doses or timing,[6,7,10] using drugs like adriamycin[5,9,10] or using associated immunotherapy.[5,10]

In May 1976 Group Inter France started a cooperative trial of adjuvant combination chemotherapy for localized breast cancer, including adriamycin followed by randomized BCG immunotherapy. Then, in May 1978 a second trial was initiated with a first randomization of chemotherapy regimen between either the same combination chemotherapy with adriamycin, or cyclophosphamide, methotrexate, 5-fluorouracil (CMF) protocol.

*Group Inter France includes the following centers participating in the trial:
Institut de Cancérologie et d'Immunogénétique, Villejuif (G. Mathé, J. L. Misset, M. Delgado, F. de Vassal); Centre Jean Perrin, Clermont-Ferrand (R. Plagne, P. Chollet, J. P. Ferriere); Centre Georges-François Leclerc, Dijon (J. Guerrin, P. Fargeot); Centre René Gauducheau, Nantes (B. Le Mevel, P. Fumoleau); CHU Bichat-Beaujon (D. Belpomme); Centre Alexis Vautrin, Nancy (R. Metz); Centre Antoine Lacassagne, Nice (M. Schneider); Centre Henri Becquerel, Rouen (C. Jeanne, M. Chevrier); Statistics Department, CHU Pitié-Salpêtrière (F. Gremy, V. Morice, J. P. Chantalou).

Patients and Methods

Patients who entered the two studies were women under 70 years of age with histologically proved breast cancer, without metastases, whose axillary nodes had been histologically studied. Good prognosis forms (T1N−), inflammatory carcinomas, and inoperable tumors were excluded.

Local treatment was modified radical mastectomy. Postoperative radiation therapy was applied or not according to the treatment protocol of each participating center.

Before entering the study and during the follow-up, the spread of disease was verified by clinical examination of chest x-ray every 3 months; skeletal scintigraphy and bone x-ray, liver scintigraphy every 6 months; carcinoembryonic antigen dosage, and liver tests every 3 months.

Combination chemotherapy was applied 2–4 weeks after surgery or after completion of radiation therapy.

In the first trial for N+ patients the chemotherapy protocol (AVCF) was as follows: day 1, adriamycin, 30 mg/m²; day 2, vincristine, 1 mg/m²; days 3–6, fluorouracil, 400 mg/m², and cyclophosphamide, 300 mg/m².

For N− patients adriamycin was excluded and the protocol (VCF) was as follows: day 1, vincristine, 1 mg/m²; days 2–6, 5-fluorouracil, 400 mg/m², and cyclophosphamide, 300 mg/m². The interval between the two cycles was 21 days

In the second trial the chemotherapy regimen was randomized between the previous protocol (AVCF for N+, VCF for N−) and CMF chemotherapy as follows: methotrexate, 40 mg/m², and 5-fluorouracil, 600 mg/m²; days 1–14, cyclophosphamide, 100 mg/m². The interval between two cycles was 14 days.

After 12 cycles, the disease-free patients were randomized to receive either BCG immunotherapy for 1 year or no further treatment.

Stratification groups were defined according to three criteria:

1. Local extent of the disease: T1T2 or T3T4
2. Nodal involvement: N− or N+
3. Pre- or postmenopausal status, menopausal status being defined as beginning at the last menstrual period plus 6 months

Patients received BCG either by scarifications or by multiple puncture gun applications at the base of each of the four limbs if the purified protein derivative (PPD) skin test had been positive and on only one limb if the test was negative, with rotation. The Pasteur immuno-BCG F was given once a week at the beginning, then spaced out according to the local reaction noted, in order to keep evolutive skin lesions permanently.

Statistical analysis was carried out using the Kaplan Meier method and the estimation of difference in probability used the Logrank test.

Results

From May 1976 until May 1978, 194 patients entered the first study. Stratification groups are indicated in Table 1. At the time of this statistical analysis (May 1981) the median follow-up time was 36 months.

After 1 year of chemotherapy, 161 patients were randomized for immunother-

Table 1. Distribution According to Stratification Criteria

	Trial 1		Trial 2	
	n	%	n	%
TXN+	5	2.6		
T1T2N+MP+	32	16.5	83	26.6
T1T2N+MP−	60	30.9	83	26.6
T2N−MP+	16	8.3	28	9
T2N−MP−	18	9.3	27	8.6
T3T4N+MP+	24	12.4	31	9.9
T3T4N+MP−	21	10.8	36	11.5
T3T4N−MP+	9	4.6	10	3.2
T3T4N−MP−	9	4.6	10	3.2
Total	194		308	

apy or no further treatment. Of these patients, 33 were excluded from randomization, 7 for relapse during chemotherapy, 21 for refusing or stopping the treatment, 5 for loss to follow-up.

Up to 1981 44 relapses and 24 deaths due to cancer were registered; 9 were local recurrences, and the others were metastatic dissemination, chiefly skeletal. These relapses appeared mainly during the second year of follow-up.

Among usual prognosis factors, the size of the tumor did not seem to influence the results, but nodal involvement remained the main factor in prognosis for disease-free survival (Fig. 1) and for overall survival. Although premenopausal women seemed to exhibit better results, the differences were not significant (Fig. 2).

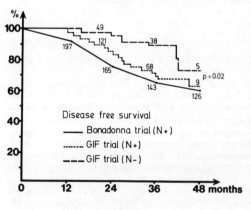

FIGURE 1.

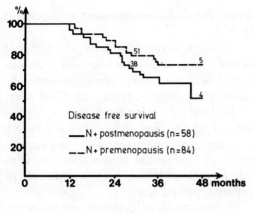

FIGURE 2.

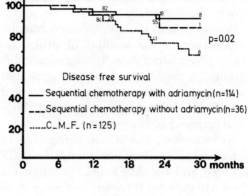

FIGURE 4.

BCG immunotherapy did not improve the results of chemotherapy: there was no significant difference between disease-free survival and overall survival (Fig. 3).

The results of the second trial are still preliminary, the average follow-up time being 20 months.

From May 1978 to 1980, 311 patients entered this study (Table 1). They were randomized to receive either VCF (38), AVCF (128), or CMF (145). After 1 year of chemotherapy, 168 were randomized for immunotherapy (87 with BCG and 81 without BCG immunotherapy).

On the whole, the same prognostic factors seemed to influence the results, especially nodal involvement. Until now, the main point of this second study appeared to be a significant difference in

disease-free survival in favor of sequential chemotherapy with adriamycin for premenopausal as well as for postmenopausal women (Fig. 4). At the time of this analysis, 33 relapses were reported: 3 for VCF protocol, 8 for AVCF, and 22 for CMF. There were 6 deaths (1 for VCF, 2 for AVCF, and 3 for CMF).

Finally, although postoperative radiotherapy was not randomized, it is interesting to observe the results of patients with nodal involvement treated with or without radiation therapy.

In the two trials, no difference in survival was seen between irradiated and nonirradiated patients (Fig. 5).

Also, the number of localized relapses was in the same range with or without radiation therapy (5/110 without radiother-

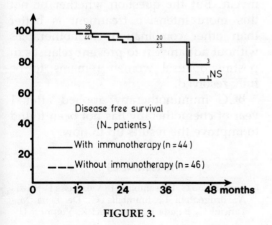

FIGURE 3.

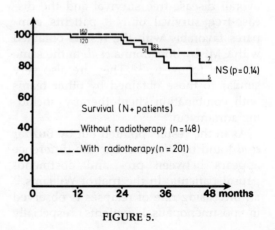

FIGURE 5.

apy and 4/84 with postoperative radiotherapy in the first trial).

Bonadonna *et al.* have pointed out the importance of the amount of drugs actually given. Until now, no significant difference in disease-free survival appeared between the patients who had received only 75% of the drugs or less and those who received 80% or more.

Nevertheless, the mean percentage of drugs actually given was higher for VCF (84.9%) and for AVCF (82.4%) than for the CMF protocol (71.9%). The mean dose of adriamycin was 85%. According to menopausal status, a significant difference ($p = 0.05$) was observed only in methotrexate doses (75% in premenopausal patients vs 64% in postmenopausal), and, finally, there was also a significant difference ($p = 0.01$) between patients who had previously received radiation therapy and those who did not receive this treatment (77% vs 84%).

The tolerance of sequential chemotherapy with adriamycin appeared to be rather good. The treatment had to be stopped for general intolerance in only 21 cases in each trial. In addition, adriamycin was discontinued in four cases in each study for minor electrocardiographic changes. No heart failure was observed.

Discussion

In these two groups of patients, the overall disease-free survival and the disease-free survival of N+ patients compares favorably with the results obtained with CMF by Bonadonna *et al.* at the same phase of follow-up.[1-3] They are also very similar to those obtained by other teams with combination chemotherapy, including adriamycin.[5,11,12]

As in the results pointed out by Buzdar *et al.*[4] and by Wendt *et al.*[10] no difference appears between pre- and postmenopausal patients. In the trial of Williams,[11] an increasing rate of relapses is observed in postmenopausal patients, especially when the nodal involvement is important ($n > 4$).

Although very preliminary, the fact that better results and better tolerance were obtained with sequential chemotherapy, including adriamycin, than with CMF must be underlined. A longer follow-up of the second trial is obviously necessary before drawing any conclusions as to the superiority of sequential chemotherapy with adriamycin in either postmenopausal or premenopausal women.

In these trials, BCG immunotherapy applied after 1 year of chemotherapy does not improve the overall results.

These findings are similar to those of Hubay and colleagues.[7]

Finally, the late effects of local treatment are also a point of discussion. The occurrence of local relapses in nonirradiated N+ patients remains until now very low, as in other trials.[3,4,6] On the other hand, a detrimental effect of radiation therapy on relapse rate seems to have occurred in the trial of Cooper and colleagues.[6] Until now, such a difference has not been found between irradiated and nonirradiated patients.

Conclusion

These preliminary results appear to be encouraging. They show a low incidence of early relapses after well-tolerated combination chemotherapy including adriamycin. But the question whether or not this more intensive treatment is better than other combination chemotherapies without adriamycin to prevent relapses in postmenopausal women remains to be fully resolved.

BCG immunotherapy applied after 1 year of chemotherapy has not been found to improve the results up to now.

REFERENCES

1. Bonadonna G, Brusamolino E, Valagussa P, Rossi A, Brugnatelli L, Brambilla C, De Lena M, Tancini G, Bajetta E, Musumeci R, Veronesi U:

Combination chemotherapy as an adjuvant treatment in operable breast cancer. *N Engl J Med 297: 405–410, 1976.*

2. Bonadonna G, Rossi A, Valagussa P, Banfi A, Veronesi U: The CMF program for operable breast cancer with positive axillary nodes: Updated analysis on the disease-free interval, site of relapse and drug tolerance. *Cancer 39: 2904–2915, 1977.*

3. Bonadonna G, Valagussa P: Dose response effect after CMF chemotherapy in breast cancer. *N Engl J Med 304: 10–15.*

4. Buzdar A, Blumenschein G, Gutterman J, Hortobagyi G, Campos L, Tashima C, Smith T, Heish E, Freirich E, Gehan E: Adjuvant therapy with 5-fluorouracil adriamycin, cyclophosphamide and BCG (FAC BCG) for stage II or III breast cancer. In *Adjuvant Therapy of Cancer II*, Jones SE, Salmon SE (Eds). Grune & Stratton, New York, 1979, pp 277–284.

5. Cooper RG, Holland JF, Glidewell O: Adjuvant chemotherapy of breast cancer. *Cancer 44: 793–798, 1979.*

6. Glucksberg H, Rivkin SE, Rasmussen S: Adjuvant chemotherapy for stage II breast cancer: A comparison of CMFPV versus L PAM. In *Adjuvant Therapy of Cancer II*, Jones SE, Salmon SE (Eds). Grune & Stratton, New York, 1979, pp 261–268.

7. Hubay CA, Pearson OH, Marshall JS, Rhodes RS, Debanne SM, Mansour EG, Hermann RE, Jones JC, Flynn WJ, Eckert C, McGuire WL: Antiestrogen, cytotoxic chemotherapy and *Bacillus* Calmette-Guerin vaccination in stage II breast cancer: A preliminary report. *Surgery 87: 494–501, 1980.*

8. Rossi A, Bonadonna G, Valagussa P, Veronesi U: Multimodal treatment in operable breast cancer: Five year results of the CMF programme. *B Med J 282: 1427–1431, 1981.*

9. Tormey D, Falkson G, Weiss R, Perloff M, Glidewell O, Holland JF: Postoperative chemotherapy with/without immunotherapy for mammary carcinoma. A preliminary report. In *Adjuvant Therapy of Cancer II*, Jones SE, Salmon SE (Eds). Grune & Stratton, New York, 1979, pp 253–260.

10. Wendt AG, Jones SE, Salmon SE, Giordano GF, Jackson RA, Miller RS, Heusinkveld RS, Moon TE: Adjuvant treatment of breast cancer with adriamycin-cyclophosphamide with or without radiation therapy. In *Adjuvant Therapy of Cancer II*, Jones SE, Salmon SE (Eds). Grune & Stratton, New York, 1979, pp 285–293.

11. Williams SD, Einborn LH, (1979): Adriamycin chemoprophylaxis of high risk breast cancer. In *Adjuvant Therapy of Cancer II*, Jones SE, Salmon SE (Eds). Grune & Stratton, New York, 1979, pp 95–301.

Part VI

Clinical Studies
New Agents

CHAPTER 21

A Phase II Study of Aclacinomycin-A in Acute Leukemia in Adults

K. Yamada, T. Nakamura, T. Tsuruo, T. Kitahara, T. Maekawa, Y. Uzuka, S. Kurita, T. Masaoka, F. Takaku, Y. Hirota, I. Amaki, S. Osamura, M. Ito, N. Nakano, M. Oguro, J. Inagaki, and K. Onozawa

Introduction

A new anthracycline antibiotic aclacinomycin A was tested for antileukemic activity and clinical toxicity in 62 patients with adult acute leukemia. The protocol was the continuous daily intravenous administration at the dose of 15 mg/m² for 7–21 days. In 21 previously untreated patients, 37% reached complete remission (CR). Five of 12 patients with acute myeloblastic leukemia, one of six with acute myelomonocytic leukemia, one of two with erythroleukemia, and the only case of acute lymphoblastic leukemia sustained CR. In 41 patients who had had prior treatment, 17% reached CR. A median total of 200 mg/m² of the drug and of 16 days of the treatment were necessary for induction of CR. Bone marrow toxicity was the major side effect.

Only one patient of the 62 had alopecia. Seven patients of the 62 showed mild electrocardiographic changes during aclacinomycin A treatment, with sinus tacycardia and flattening or inversion of T waves. The alterations were completely restored during continuation of the drug in five patients and 2–3 days after cessation of the treatment in two patients. None of the patients developed signs of congestive heart failure or of cardiomyopathy.

The established therapeutic effectiveness comparable to that of daunorubicin and adriamycin, and the least cardiac and alopecic toxicity, indicate that aclacinomycin A deserves further clinical trials for phase III study in acute leukemia as well as for phase II–III study in malignant lymphoma.

Aclacinomycin A (ACM) is a new anthracycline antibiotic isolated from *Streptomyces galilaeus* by Oki et al.[10,11] It consists of the tetracyclic quinoid aglycone aklavinone linked to the amino sugar L-rhodosamine and to two other deoxysugars, 2-deoxy-L-fucose and L-cinerulose A (Fig. 1).

The compound has shown wide antitumor activity against ascitic and solid forms of various experimental tumors,[5,11] including L1210 and P388 leukemias, and B16 melanoma. The antitumor activity of ACM in L1210 and P388 leukemias was comparable to that of daunorubicin (DNR), but at two times the dose level of adriamycin (ADM). Animal toxicology[5,10] showed that the LD_{50} of ACM was two to three times as high as that of DNR and ADM, and both acute and subacute cardiotoxicity of ACM, measured in terms of electrocardiogram (ECG) patterns and histologic and electron microscopic changes of the myocardium, was far less than that of ADM.[3,15] ACM showed a greater inhibition effect on RNA synthesis than did

First Department of Internal Medicine, Nagoya University School of Medicine, Japan

137

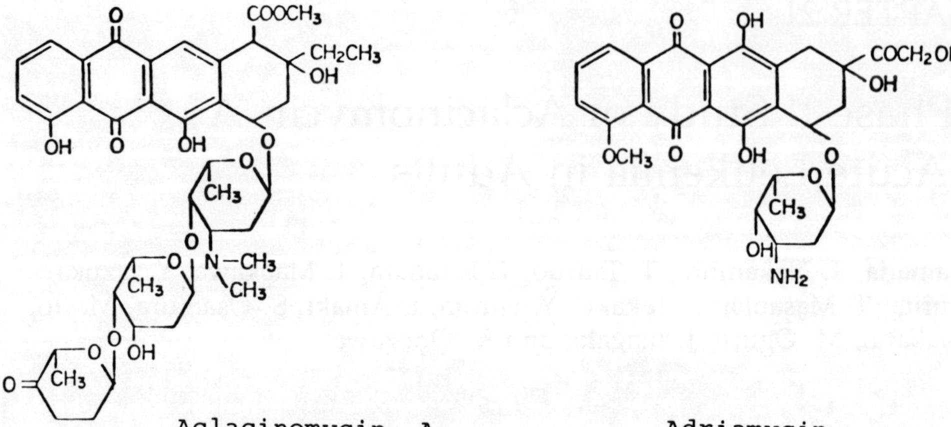

Aclacinomycin A   Adriamycin

FIGURE 1.   Chemical structure of aclacinomycin A and adriamycin.

DNR and ADM,[2,11] and it has no mutagenic activity, although DNR and ADM are highly mutagenic.[14]

Hence, after phase I trials in man,[4,8,9,12,13,17] a phase II study of ACM in adult patients with acute leukemia was conducted by a Cooperative Study Group on the Treatment of Leukemia by Grant-in-Aid for Cancer Research from the Ministry of Health and Welfare of Japan.

Materials and Methods

All adults with acute leukemia were eligible for inclusion in the study, regardless of morphologic type, clinical status, or other considerations. ACM was supplied by the Sanraku-Ocean Co. Ltd. (Tokyo) in a 20-mg vial. It was dissolved in 500 ml of physiologic saline and was administered intravenously for 1 hour. The protocol chosen for leukemia was the continuous daily administration at the dose of 15 mg/m²/day. The aim throughout was to continue drug administration during the induction phase to the point of the maximum tolerable amount, which would, it was hoped, result in a hypoplastic marrow or complete remission (CR). Throughout the study, supportive therapy, including leukocyte and platelet transfusion, was

used when indicated. Evaluation during the study included the monitoring of hematologic values, hepatic and renal functions, and ECG. CR was defined as a state of less than 5% blasts in the bone marrow nuclear cells and normal hematopoietic components, as well as no signs attributable to leukemia. In the results to be discussed, only CR is considered significant.

Blood level and urinary excretion of ACM and its metabolites were determined in patients by the thin-layer chromatography-fluorescence method.

Results

Of the 62 adult patients with acute leukemia, 41 had had prior treatment with chemotherapy and 21 were previously untreated. There were 37 males and 25 females, with a mean age of 39 years, ranging from 15 to 81 years.

Of the 21 previously untreated patients, 38% responded with CR (Table 1). There were 5 CRs in 12 patients with acute myelogenous leukemia, 1 CR in 6 patients with acute myelomonocytic leukemia, 1 CR in 2 patients with erythroleukemia, and the only patient with acute lymphoblastic leukemia had CR. Of the 41 patients

Table 1. Phase II Study of Aclacinomycin A in Acute Leukemia—Previously Untreated Patients

Type[a]	No. of Patients	CR	PR[b]	F[c]	CR Rate (%)
AML	12	5	0	7	41.7
AMoL	6	1	2	3	16.7
EL	2	1	0	1	50.0
ALL	1	1	0	0	100.0
Total	21	8	2	11	38.0

[a] AML: acute myelogenous leukemia; AMoL: acute myelomonocytic leukemia; EL: erythroleukemia; ALL: acute lymphoblastic leukemia.
[b] PR: partial response.
[c] F: failure.

Table 2. Phase II Study of Aclacinomycin A in Acute Leukemia—Previously Treated Patients

Type[a]	No. of Patients	CR	PR[b]	F[c]	CR Rate (%)
AML	24	4	5	15	16.7
AMoL	7	0	1	6	0
AProL	2	2	0	0	100.0
ALL	8	1	0	7	12.5
Total	41	7	6	28	17.0

[a] AML: acute myelogenous leukemia; AMoL: acute myelomonocytic leukemia; ALL: acute lymphoblastic leukemia.
[b] PR: partial response.
[c] F: failure.

who had prior treatment with chemotherapy, 17% responded with CR (Table 2). Thus responses with CR were noted with an overall rate of 24.2%.

A median total of 200 mg/m² with a range of 93–275 mg/m² and a median total of 16 days with a range of 7–21 days were necessary for induction of CR. As shown in Table 3, in a group of patients who received a total dose of not more than 200 mg, the CR rate was only 9.1%, yet it increased to a level of 26–28% in those receiving 201–300 mg or in those with more than 301 mg in total.

Toxicity

The incidence and degree of drug toxicity were measured during and after the study, the predominant effects being those related to marrow depression (Table 3). The nadir of the peripheral leukocyte ranged from 200 to 6700/cm with a median of 1200/cm, which was reached on the 20th median day. The nadir of the platelet ranged from 2000 to 46,000/cm, with a median of 9000/cm, being reached on the 18th median day. Hematuria (13%) and tarry stool (5%) were noted. The gastrointestinal effects were seen in nausea and vomiting (38%), anorexia (32%), and diarrhea (12%), as well as such other side effects as stomatitis (15%) and phlebitis (10%).

Liver impairment with elevation of alkaline phosphatase, GOT, and GPT were found in 6% of the patients. In most of these, hepatic enzymes returned to normal level after cessation of treatment. It is to be emphasized that only 1 of the 62 patients had alopecia. ECG changes were recorded in 7 (11%) of the 62 patients. The abnormalities noted in these patients were sinus tachycardia and flattening or inversion of the T wave. In five cases, the changes were transient and the drug administration was continued. In two cases, in whom administration of the drug was discontinued, the observed alterations were completely restored.

Clinical Pharmacology

The plasma disappearance curve of ACM and its metabolites in three patients after a single intravenous injection of 25 mg/m² of the drug was studied. The curve is biphasic; the half-life of the initial phase is 30 minutes and that of the second phase is 120 minutes. At 20 minutes after the injection, the ACM level is maximum at 26 ng/ml, and falls exponentially to zero by 8 hours. The active metabolites of ACM, MA144 M1 and MA144 N1, rose for the first 4 hours; the plateau was reached at the level of 10 ng/ml, and then gradually decreased over a period of 24 hours. The urinary excretion pattern of ACM and the

Table 3. Side Effects in 62 Cases of Aclacinomycin A Treatment—Acute Leukemia

Side Effect	Rate (%)
Nausea and vomiting	38
Anorexia	32
Stomatitis	15
Hematuria	13
Diarrhea	12
Phlebitis	10
Hepatic dysfunction	6
Tarry stool	5
Renal dysfunction	3
Precordial oppression	3
Alopecia	1
Changes of ECG	16.6

metabolites in seven patients is as follows. In 24 hours, about 6% of the dose was excreted; 0.6% was ACM, 4.6%, active metabolites, and 0.9%, inactive metabolites.

Discussion

ACM was tested for antitumor activity and clinical toxicity in 62 adult patients with acute leukemia. The observed CR rate of 38% in the previously untreated patients is comparable to that reported for ADM and DNR with the various dose regimens.[16,17] The CR rate of 17% in the previously untreated patients is encouraging because most of the respondents were considered to be resistant to either DNR or ADM. In fact, there are some patients who had CR to ACM after completely failing to respond to an adequate trial of DNR or ADM. This evidence lends credence to the contention that ACM is not necessarily cross-resistant with either DNR or ADM, although animal experiments using DNR-resistant L1210 and ADM-resistant P388 leukemias indicated that ACM had cross-resistance to both agents.[5,11]

The major limiting factors for the use of either DNR or ADM are alopecia and cardiotoxicity. In our series of patients only 1 of 62 patients had alopecia. Mathé et al.[7] reported no hair loss in any of the 12 patients in their phase II study of ACM. Danchev et al.[3] systematically submitted

all anthracycline analogues to electron microscopic study of the myocardium of golden hamsters and reported that ACM was the least cardiotoxic. Hori et al.[5] and Wakabayashi et al.[15] reported that cardiotoxicity of ACM in rabbits and hamsters was less than one-fifteenth of that of ADM. In our clinical studies, 11% of the 62 patients showed such ECG changes as tachycardia or ST-T abnormalities, but in every case the alterations completely reversed to normal during continuation or after cessation of the treatment. No one had clinical signs of congestive heart failure attributable to ACM treatment. Mathé also reported that only 1 of the 20 patients in whom the effect of ACM on the heart was evaluable presented a cardiac intolerance with negative T waves after a total dose of 42 mg, which became normal after discontinuation of the drug. Yamagata et al.[18] reported that palpitation and sinus tachycardia were seen in three patients who received a cumulative ACM dose of 1000 mg. Oka[9] reported ECG changes in 10 of the 197 patients in a phase I–II study of ACM. A recent survey of cardiotoxicity in the Cooperative Group Study on ACM showed that ECG changes were recorded in 18 (6%) of the 270 patients in whom ECG was monitored during the treatment.[1] A variety of changes, such as tachycardia, atrial fibrillation, low voltage, ST-T changes, and unspecified arrhythmia during ACM treatment are considered nonspecific, occurring at various dose levels irrespective of dosage schedule. There was no clinical sign of congestive heart failure or that of cardiomyopathy, even in a group of 40 patients who received a cumulative dose of ACM of 500 mg/m². Thus it was estimated that clinical cardiotoxicity of ACM appears to be much less than that reported for ADM and DNR.[6]

In our clinical pharmacology study of ACM, the plasma levels declined rapidly after intravenous administration, suggesting rapid uptake into tissues. In the meantime, rapid elevation and long persistence of the active metabolites indicate that enzymatic keto reduction to the pharmacologically active products MA144 M1 and MA144 N1 is the major step in biotransformation.

Ogawa et al.[8] reported objective responses in patients with malignant lymphoma in their phase I study of ACM. A recent survey of ACM efficacy in the treatment of non-Hodgkin's lymphoma showed that of the 29 patients, 17% responded with CR and 34% with partial remission.[1]

It has been established that the therapeutic effectiveness of ACM is comparable to DNR and ADM and that ACM is the least cardiotoxic and alopecic. These findings indicate that ACM deserves further clinical trials for phase III study in acute leukemia as well as for phase II–III study in malignant lymphoma. Such studies are now under way.

ACKNOWLEDGMENTS

This investigation was supported by a Grant-in Aid for Cancer Research from the Ministry of Health and Welfare (Grant No. 54-5) under the title of "Multidisciplinary Studies on the Treatment of Leukemia."

We gratefully acknowledge the support of Sanraku Ocean Co. Ltd. in supplying the aclacinomycin A used in this study, and Dr. H. Umezawa and Dr. T. Oki in supplying the experimental data as well as precious advice on which these studies were based.

REFERENCES

1. Cooperative Group Study in Aclacinomycin A. Interim Report Part 6, 1980.
2. Crooke SP, Duvernay, VH, Galvan L, Prestayko AW: Structural activity relationship to effect on macromolecular synthesis. Mol Pharmacol 14: 290–298, 1978.
3. Dantchev D, Slioussartchoùk V, Paintrand M, Hayat M, Bourat C, Mathé G: Electron microscopic studies of the heart and light microsopic studies of the skin after treatment of golden hamsters with adriamycin, detorubicin, AD-32, and aclacinomycin. Cancer Treat Rep 63: 875–888, 1979.
4. Furue H, Komita T, Nakao I, Furukawa I, Kanko T, Yokoyama T: Clinical experiences with aclacinomycin A. Recent Results Cancer Res 63: 242–246, 1978.
5. Hori S, Shirai M, Hirano S, Oki T, Inui T, Tukagoshi S, Ishizuka M, Takeuchi T, Umezawa H: Antitumor activity of new anthracycline antibiotics, aclacinomycin-A and its analogs, and their toxicity. Gan 68: 685–690, 1977.
6. Lenaz L, Pagae JA: Cardiotoxicity of adriamycin and related anthracyclines. Cancer Treat Rev 3: 111–120, 1976.
7. Mathé G, Bayssas M, Gouveia J, Danchec D, Ribaud P, Machover D, Misset J, Schwarlenberg L, Jasmin C, Hayat M: Preliminary results of a phase II trial of aclacinomycin in acute leukemia and lymphosarcoma. Cancer Chemother Pharmacol 1: 259–262, 1978.
8. Ogawa M, Inagaki J, Horikoshi N, Inoue K, Chinen T, Ueoka H, Nagura E: Clinical study of aclacinomycin A. Cancer Treat Rep 63: 931–934, 1979.
9. Oka S: A review of clinical studies on aclacinomycin A — phase I and preliminary phase II evaluation of ACM-A. Sci Rep Res Inst Tohoku Univ 25: 37–49, 1978.
10. Oki T, Matsuzawa Y, Yoshimoto A, Numata K, Kitamura I, Hori S, Takamatasu A, Umezawa H, Ishizuka M, Naganawa H, Suda H, Hamada M, Takeuchi T: New antitumor antibiotics, aclacinomycin A and B. J Antibiot (Tokyo) 28: 830–834, 1975.
11. Oki T: A new anthracycline antibiotic. Jpn J Antibiot 30 Suppl: 70–84, 1977.
12. Sakano T, Okazaki N, Ise T, Kitaoka K, Kimura K: Phase I study of aclacinomycin A. Jpn J Clin Oncol 8: 49–53, 1978.
13. Suzuki H, Kawashima K, Yamada K: Aclacinomycin A, a new antileukemic agent. Lancet 1: 870–871, 1979.
14. Umezawa K, Sawamura M, Matsushima T, Sugimura T: Mutagenicity of aclacinomycin A and daunomycin derivatives. Cancer Res 38: 1782–1874, 1978.
15. Wakabayashi T, Oki T, Tone H, Hirano S, Omori K: A comparative electron microscopic study of aclacinomycin and adriamycin cardiotoxicities in rabbits and hamsters. J Electron Microsc (Tokyo) 29: 106–118, 1980.
16. Weil M, Glidewell J, Jacquillat C, Levy R, Serpick A, Wiernick PH, Oliver J et al.: Daunorubicin in the therapy of acute granulocytic leukemia. Cancer Res 33: 921–928, 1973.
17. Wiernik PH: Use of adriamycin (NSC-123127) in hematologic malignancies. Cancer Chemother Rep 3: 369–373, 1975.
18. Yamagata S, Niimoto M, Hamai Y, Hattori T: Clinical study of aclacinomycin A. (Abstract) In Proceedings of the 26th Annual Meeting of Chemotherapy. Tokyo, 1978, p. 137.

CHAPTER 22

Phase II Clinical Trial of Aclacinomycin-A in Acute Leukemia and Leukemic Non-Hodgkin Lymphoma

G. Mathé, R. De Jager, M. Delgado, D. Machover, P. Ribaud, F. De Vassal,
M. Gil-Delgado, J. L. Misset, J. Gouveia, C. Jasmin, M. Hayat, J. Gastiaburu,
L. Schwarzenberg[a], R. Hulhoven, P. Michaux, G. Sokal[b]

Aclacinomycin A (ACM) is an anthracycline produced by fermentation of *Streptomyces galileus* MA144-MI.[1] Structural differences between adriamycin (ADM) and ACM involve the phenolic groups and the ring substituants, including the number and the structure of the sugars (Fig. 1). ACM is an intercalating agent, as are the other anthracyclines, but unlike ADM, which inhibits DNA and RNA syntheses equally, ACM inhibits RNA much more than DNA synthesis.[2] ACM is metabolized by the liver in cytotoxic glycosides and inactive aglycones. The cytotoxic glycosides are themselves inactivated by microsomal reduction.[3]

We selected ACM from several anthracyclines showing antitumor activity in experimental tumor systems[4] for clinical trial because Dantchev *et al.*[5] have demonstrated that ACM in the golden hamster model did not cause alopecia or significant cardiotoxicity. AD-32 was the only other anthracycline to yield only minimal cardiotoxicity in this model. Experimentally, we have observed that ACM does not induce immunosuppression but that it tends to stimulate immune reactions *stricto et lato sensu*.[6] Finally, ACM was not mutagenic in the standard testing systems,[7,8] which for an anthracycline is quite exceptional.

Following the results of phase I studies conducted in Japan,[9] we chose to administer ACM at the dose of 10–30 mg/m² for 10–30 days, depending on therapeutic efficacy and tolerance. Favorable results were obtained, but at the cost of marked intestinal toxicity.[10] Therefore in an attempt to decrease toxicity while keeping the same level of therapeutic activity, we modified the administration schedule as follows: ACM 15 mg/m²/day for 10 days, to be repeated two or more times and leaving a rest period of 10 days between courses.

The purpose of this chapter is to analyze the data concerning the activity and toxicity of ACM observed during the two segments of the phase II trial in patients with acute leukemia and leukemic lymphosarcoma (LSL).

Patients and Methods

PHASE IIA TRIAL IN ACUTE LEUKEMIA AND LEUKEMIC LYMPHOSARCOMA

From September 1977 to August 1980, 50 patients were admitted to the study, 45 were evaluable for toxicity and therapeutic efficacy.

All patients had received prior treatment with one or more conventional chemother-

[a]Institut de Cancérologie et d'Immunogénétique (INSERM U-50), de l'Hôpital Universitaire Paul-Brousse, Villejuif, France
[b]Hôpital Saint Luc, U.C.L., Bruxelles, Belgique

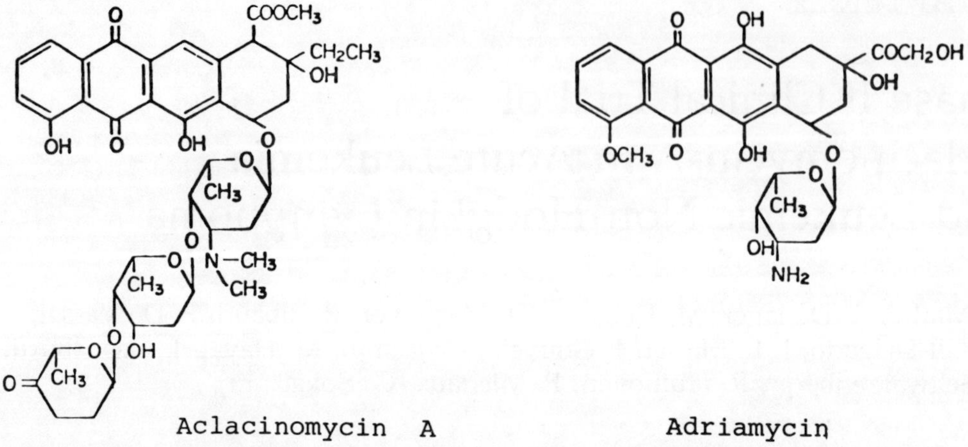

Aclacinomycin A   Adriamycin

FIGURE 1.   Chemical structure of aclacinomycin A and adriamycin.

apy regimens. Eleven patients with acute myelogenous leukemia (AML) were considered resistant to ADM, which they had received along with vincristine (VCR) and cytosine arabinoside (Ara-C). Resistance was either primary or secondary.

The 19 patients with acute lymphoblastic leukemia (ALL) had benefited from 1–7 prior remissions induced by ADM combined with VCR, prednisone, and asparaginase. No attempt was made to reinduce them with the same combination prior to receiving ACM. Their status in terms of ADM resistance is therefore unknown. The same is true for the 11 LSL patients.

Patients received 10–30 mg/m² of ACM as a slow I.V. infusion for 10–30 days, depending on tolerance.

PHASE IIB TRIAL IN ACUTE MYELOID LEUKEMIA

This segment of the study from August 1980 to May 1981, was restricted to acute myeloid leukemia (AML) patients. Of 22 patients evaluable as of May 1981, 17 presented with AML, 2 with acute myelomonocytic leukemia, and 3 with oligoblastic leukemia.

They received the following protocol treatment: ACM, 15 mg/m²/day I.V. for 10 days followed by a 10-day rest period. These 10-day cycles were repeated two or more times until remission induction.

EVALUATION OF TREATMENT AND FOLLOW-UP

Daily blood counts were obtained for all patients. Bone marrow aspirations were performed at least once a week. Hepatic and renal function tests and blood electrolytes were done twice a week. Whenever severe pancytopenia secondary to bone marrow aplasia occurred, patients were taken to sterile rooms[11] for intensive care, including leukocyte[12] and/or platelet transfusions and antibiotics.[13] Complete remission (CR) was defined as a treatment-inducing M1 bone marrow: <5% blasts with normal cellularity, peripheral blood counts with >10³/mm³ neutrophils and >10⁵/mm³ platelets. Partial remission (PR) was defined as a 50% reduction in the percentage of blasts in the bone marrow with enough recovery of normal cellularity to maintain >10³/mm³ neutrophils and >10⁵/mm³ platelets (M2 bone marrow). The duration of remission is not a useful parameter in this study, since patients received maintenance therapy after achieving CR. Failure of treatment or M3 marrow corresponds to the persistence of >50% blasts in a marrow showing poor cellularity.

Results

PHASE IIA IN AML, ALL, AND LNHL

Remission induction and dose correlation

Patients' characteristics prior to treatment are given in Table 1 and results in Table 2. Of 17 patients with AML, 4 CR and 5 PR were obtained. CR was obtained only in patients having received a cumulative ACM dose ≥300 mg/m². PR was observed in two of seven patients at ACM doses ≥300 mg/m² and in three of ten at a dose of less than 300 mg/m².

The results in ALL suggest a similar dose dependency but two CRs were documented at cumulative doses of less than 300 mg/m².

In LNHL, two CR and three PR were obtained at total ACM doses between 199 and 299 mg/m². The cumulative ACM dose was the only significant parameter correlated with remission induction in AML. Other factors such as age, percent of bone marrow blasts prior to treatment, and the number of prior remissions, were not statistically significant.

The duration of remission cannot be directly attributed to ACM induction, since all patients subsequently received maintenance chemotherapy with other drugs. It should, however, be stressed that among 11 AML patients clinically resistant to ADM, i.e., resistant to reinduction with VCR, ADM, and Ara-C, 4 CR and 2 PR were obtained with ACM (Table 3).

Toxicity

All responding patients presented severe myelosuppression. Despite intensive care in a microbiologically controlled room,[11] leukocyte[12] and/or platelet transfusions,[13] and antibiotics, four patients died with bone marrow aplasia. Diarrhea was the major nonhematologic toxicity. Severe, occasionally hemorrhagic, diarrhea occurred in all patients after more than 10 days of ACM treatment. This observation led us to design empirically the 10-day administration cycles used in the second segment of the study.

Nausea and/or vomiting and stomatitis occurred in 37% of the cases. Minor electrocardiographic (ECG) alterations (ST-T wave abnormalities) were seen in 13%. Hair loss attributable to ACM was not seen in patients who were not alopecic from

Table 1. Characteristics of Patients

Tumor Type	No. of Patients	No. of Evaluable Patients	Sex (M/F)	Age (Median and Extremes)	No. of Prior Remissions	No. of Patients
AML	20	17	12/5	25 (14–56)	0	4
					1	7
					2	5
					3	1
ALL	19	19	13/6	12 (3–47)	1	4
					2	9
					3	4
					4	1
					7	1
LNHL	11	8	7/1	19 (7–49)	0	4
					1	3
					3	1

Table 2. Correlation Between the Total Dose and Effect

Tumor Type	Total Dose (mg/m^2)	No. of Evaluable Patients	Therapeutic Effect CR	PR	CR + PR	Failure
AML	100–199	6	0	1		5
	200–299	4	0	2		2
	300–412	7	4	2		1
ALL	60–199	9	1	0		2
	199–299	8	1	1		6
	300–412	2	0	1		1
LNHL	90–199	3	0	0		3
	199–299	5	2	1		2
Total of primary leukemias and LSL		45	8 + 2[a]	8	16[a]	23
Total of trials in primary leukemias and LSL		47	10	8	18	25

[a]One AML patient and one LSL patient have achieved a second CR with ACM after relapsing during maintenance therapy without ACM.

prior treatment. There were no hepatic or renal toxicities recorded.

PHASE IIB IN AML

Therapeutic activity

Of 26 patients admitted to the study as of May 1981, 22 were evaluable for therapeutic activity. CR was obtained in nine patients (41%) and PR in two patients (9%). Patients with oligoblastic leukemia did not achieve remissions. CR was achieved in three patients after a total ACM dose of 150 mg/m^2 (one cycle), in four patients after 300 mg/m^2 (two cycles), and in two patients at 450 mg/m^2 (three cycles). These results confirm the dose-dependent therapeutic activity of ACM in AML.

Table 3. Complete and Partial Remissions in Acute Myeloid Leukemia Resistant to ADM

	ADM[a] Resistance Known	Unknown
No. of patients	11	6
CR	4	–
PR	2	3
Failures	5	3

[a]ADM administered in combination with VCR and Ara-C.

All patients were pretreated with combination chemotherapy, including daunorubicin (DNR) or ADM. The lack of clinical cross-resistance between DNR/ADM and ACM is confirmed by the fact that five CR were documented in eight patients showing primary or secondary resistance to chemotherapy regimens, including one anthracycline.

Toxicity

All 22 patients presented severe myelosuppression. Death during bone marrow aplasia occurred in four cases: three patients dying from uncontrolled pneumonia and septicemia and one patient from a cerebral hemorrhage.

Diarrhea, including one case of pseudomembranous colitis, occurred only in 2 of 22 (nearly 10%) patients.

Acute reversible ECG changes (ST-T wave abnormalities) were seen in two patients. Echocardiographic control was normal in both cases.

In these series of patients, three cases of transient hepatic dysfunction that could be drug-related were recorded. There was no abnormality of renal function and no patients (who could be evaluated for alopecia) presented alopecia secondary to ACM treatment.

Discussion

ACM, as published in our preliminary reports in 1978[10] and 1979[14], is a drug capable of inducing CR and PR in AML, ALL, and LNHL.

Remission induction appears clearly dose-dependent in AML, most CR occurring at cumulative doses of ACM $\geqslant 300$ mg/m^2. The same probably holds true for ALL and LNHL, although remissions were seen at lower doses than with AML. Further data are needed to elucidate this point in these neoplasias. This is especially important for NHL, a disease for which few active drugs exist.[15]

The 4% CR rate (9 of 22) observed in AML in the second part of the study is quite remarkable in this heavily pretreated group of patients. Furthermore, ACM is of great interest, because it appears active against AML that is clinically resistant to combination chemotherapy including ADM which was not predicted by the experimental results obtained with L1210/ADM.[16] A similar discrepancy between clinical results[17,18] and experimental data was observed for the Vinca Alkaloids: patients considered clinically resistant to VCR responded to vindesine as well.[19]

Finally, the absence of hair loss predicted by the hamster model[5] as well as the low cardiotoxicity and lack of mutagenicity,[8] add to the interest of this new agent.

The severe diarrhea that was prevalent in the first part of our study was almost completely eliminated by schedule manipulation.

ACM appears to be a new major drug for remission induction in AML. The apparent lack of cross-resistance between ACM and ADM combination chemotherapy makes the drug especially attractive for the treatment of a disease for which, despite high remission induction rates, the median survival remains short.

Our results and efficacy of ACM in AML have been confirmed by the Japanese Cooperative Study Group on the Treatment of Leukemia.[20]

REFERENCES

1. Oki T, Matsuzawa Y, Yoshimoto A, Numata K, Kimatura I, Ori S, Takamatsu A, Umezawa H, Ishizuka M, Naganawa H, Suda H, Hamada M, Takeuchi T: New antitumor antibiotics aclacinomycins A and B. *Jpn J Antibiot 28: 830–834, 1975.*
2. Oki T: New anthracycline antibiotics. *Jpn J Antibiot 30 Suppl: 570–584, 1977.*
3. Komiyama T, Oki T, Inui T, Takeuchi T, Umezawa H: Reduction of anthracycline glycoside by NADPH-cytochrome P-450 reductase. *Gan 70: 403–410, 1979.*
4. Mathé G, De Jager R, Maral R (Eds): *Anthracyclines.* Current Status and future developments. Masson, New York, 1983.
5. Dantchev D, Slioussartchouck V, Paintrand M, Hayat M, Bourut C, Mathé G: Electron microscopy studies of the heart and light microscopic studies of the skin after treatment of golden hamsters with adriamycin, detorubicin, AD-32 and aclacinomycin. *Cancer Treat Rep 63: 875–888, 1979.*
6. Orbach-Arbouys S, Andrade-Mena CE, Berardet M, Mathé G: Potentiated immune responses after administration of aclacinomycin. In preparation.
7. Umezawa H, Sawamura M, Matsushima T, Sugimura T: Mutagenicity of aclacinomycin-A and daunomycin derivatives. *Cancer Res 38: 1782–1784, 1980.*
8. Marzin D, Jasmin C, Maral R, Mathé G: Mutagenicity in five strains of Salmonella typhimurium of seven anthracycline derivatives. Submitted for publication in *Cancer Res,* 1982.
9. Furue H, Komita T, Nakao I, Furukawa I, Kanko T, Yokoyama T: Clinical experiences with aclacinomycin. In *Antitumor Antibiotics,* Carter SK, Umezawa H, Douros J, Sakurai Y (Eds). Springer-Verlag, New York, 1978, pp 241–246.
10. Mathé G, Bayssas M, Gouveia J, Dantchev D, Ribaud P, Machover D, Misset JL, Schwarzenberg L, Jasmin C, Hayat M: Preliminary results of a phase II trial of aclacinomycin in acute leukemia and lymphosarcoma. *Cancer Chemother Pharmacol 1: 259–262, 1978.*
11. Mathé G, Forestier P: Un outil moderne de la recherche médicale: l'Institut de Cancérologie et d'Immunogénétique. Intrication de la recherche expérimentale et clinique, conditionnement hyposeptique des animaux et des malades. *Techn Hosp 20: 47–49, 1965.*
12. Schwarzenberg L, Cattan A, Schneider M, Schlumberger JR, Amiel JL, Mathé G: La réanimation hématologique II. Correction des désordres graves des leucocytes et des immunoglobulines. *Presse Med 74: 1061–1065, 1966.*
13. Schwarzenberg L, Cattan A, Schneider M, Schlumberger JR, Amiel JL, Mathé G: La réanimation hématologique. I. Correction des désordres graves de la lignée érythrocytaire et des désordres de la coagulation. *Presse Med 74: 969–972, 1966.*
14. Mathé G, Gil MA, Gescher F, Delgado M, Bayssas M, Ribaud P, Misset JL, Hayat M, Machover D: Aclacinomycin in acute leukaemias and lymphomas. *Lancet 2: 310–311, 1979.*

15. Mathé G, Belpomme D, Dantchev D, Khalil A, Afifi AM, Taleb N, Pouillart P, Schwarzenberg L, Hayat M, De Vassal F, Jasmin C, Misset JL, Musset M: Immunoblastic lymphosarcomas: cytological and clinical entity? *Biomedicine 22: 473–488, 1975*.

16. Maral R, Bourut C, Chenu E, Mathé G: Experimental *in vivo* cross-resistance of two anthracyclines. *Cancer Lett (In press)*.

17. Mathé G, Misset JL, De Vassal F, Hayat M, Gouveia J, Machover D, Belpomme D, Schwarzenberg L, Ribaud P, Pico JL, Musset M, Jasmin C, De Luca L: Traitement de leucémies et hématosarcomes par la vindésine. Résultats d'un essai phase II en termes d'induction de rémission. *Nouv Presse Med 7: 525–528, 1978*.

18. Bayssas M, Gouveia J, Ribaud P, Musset M, De Vassal F, Pico JL, De Luca L, Misset JL, Machover D, Belpomme D, Schwarzenberg L, Jasmin C, Hayat M, Mathé G: Phase II-trial with vindesine for regression induction in patients with leukemias and hematosarcomas. *Cancer Chemother Pharmacol 2: 247–255, 1979*.

19. Maral R, Bourut C, Chenu E, Mathé G: Experimental *in vivo* cross-resistance of vinca alkaloid drugs. *Cancer Chemother Pharmacol 5: 197–200, 1981*.

20. Yamada K, Nakamura T, Tsuruo T, Kitahara T, Maekawa T, Uzaka Y, Kurita S, Masaoka T, Takaku F, Hirota Y, Amaki I, Osamura S, Ito M, Nakano M, Oguro M, Inagaki J, Unozawa K: A phase II study of aclacinomycin-A in acute leukemia in adults. *Cancer Treat Rev 7: 177–182, 1980*.

CHAPTER 23

Toxic and Therapeutic Activity of 4'-Epidoxorubicin

V. Bonfante

4'-Epidoxorubicin (4'-epi-DOX) is a doxorubicin (DOX) analogue compound developed with the attempt to improve the therapeutic index of the anthracycline antibiotics. It was obtained by modification of the natural amino sugar daunosamine (3-amino-2,3,6-trideoxy-L-lyxohexose), which is replaced by the corresponding 4'-epi-analogue (3-amino-2,3,6-trideoxy-L-arabinohexose).[1]

In experimental studies, the antitumor activity of 4'-epi-DOX was shown to be equal to that of DOX. General toxicity and cardiac toxicity were lower compared to that of DOX when 4'-epi-DOX was tested in mice and rabbits during acute and chronic toxicity studies.[2] Therefore 4'-epi-DOX showed an increased therapeutic ratio and was considered a compound worthy of clinical trial, which began at the Istituto Nazionale Tumori in July 1977. Preliminary results were reported in two previous publications.[3,4] In this chapter we analyze the experience achieved with 108 patients entered in phase I and II study.

Patients and Methods

PATIENT SELECTION

All patients who were included in the study had histologic confirmation of a malignant disease, which had become refractory to conventional pharmacologic treatments or for which there was no therapy of proven clinical benefit. No patient

Istituto Nazionale Tumori, Milan, Italy

had received chemotherapy and/or radiotherapy within the preceding 3 weeks.

Pretreatment evaluation consisted of a complete medical history and physical examination. Laboratory evaluation included complete hemogram and biochemical profile. Chest x-ray was obtained in all patients. Additional radiologic and scintigraphic studies were performed only when indicated by the clinical situation. Follow-up studies included weekly complete hemograms; patients were followed closely for any evidence of toxicity and appropriate roentgenographic studies were repeated prior to every course to document drug response. Cardiologic evaluation consisted of the systematic recording of arterial blood pressure, pulse rate, electrocardiogram (ECG), and left ventricular systolic time intervals determined according to the method described by Weissler et al.[5]

DRUG ADMINISTRATION

4'-Epi-DOX was administered by rapid intravenous injection every 3 weeks. The starting dose level was 10 mg/m^2; progressive dose escalation was carried out according to the Fibonacci scheme up to the dose of 50 mg/m^2. Subsequently, we selected doses (60–75 and 90 mg/m^2) that could be comparable to therapeutically effective doses of DOX. Therapy was discontinued if disease progression became evident or when the total dose of 4'-epi-DOX, including that of prior DOX in eight patients was approaching 550 mg/m^2.

PATIENT CHARACTERISTICS

The 108 patients who entered into the study (61 males and 47 females) had a median age of 50 years (18–73 years). The 99 patients who received a total of 342 cycles of 4'-epi-DOX had adequate trial. Nine patients were considered unevaluable either because of early death due to progressive cancer, not related to drug toxicity (6 patients), or loss to follow-up (3 patients). Prior therapy included conventional chemotherapy in 52 patients, radiation therapy in 13 patients, and both modalities in 17 patients. In particular, 8 patients also had received DOX to a mean total dose of 200 mg/m² (range, 60–320 mg/m²). Twenty-six patients had been previously untreated.

Results

TOXICITY

The toxic manifestations observed with 4'-epi-DOX are summarized in Table 1. The pattern of side effcts was equal to that observed after DOX. However, gastrointestinal and hematologic toxicity were less severe than those seen at comparable doses of doxorubicin.

Acute cardiac toxicity of 4'-epi-DOX was detected by ECG abnormalities that were characterized by arrhythmias, in particular ventricular premature contractions and nonspecific changes of ST-T wave. The variation of PEP/LVET ratio expressed as a percent change (+Δ%) from basal values, produced by different single doses of 4'-epi-DOX in comparison with DOX, is illustrated in Figure 1. Both drugs induced a dose-dependent decrease of left ventricular function as measured by PEP/LVET ratio. However, the 4'-epi-DOX curve is shifted to the right, thus indicating a lower toxic effect on myocardial contractility compared with DOX. Chronic cardiac toxicity of 4'-epi-DOX was monitored by systolic time intervals measured after different cumulative doses in 14 patients who

Table 1. Percent Toxic Manifestations

	Patients			
	6 (50 mg/ m²)	31 (60 mg/ m²)	31 (75 mg/ m²)	35 (90 mg/ m²)
Nausea	66	70	55	71
Vomiting	33	48	42	46
Stomatitis			9	5
Diarrhea				5
Fever >38°C			9	5
Alopecia	66	52	77	80
Leukopenia[a]				
Total	66	52	55	51
Untreated	100	100	60	36
Previous RT[b]	100	33	100	83
Previous CH[b] ± RT	50	46	41	50
Thrombocytopenia[c]				
Total	50	16	13	6
Untreated		25	10	9
Previous RT		33	25	
Previous CH ± RT	75	12	12	11

[a]Leukocytes <4000/mm³.
[b]CH: chemotherapy; RT: radiotherapy.
[c]Platelets <110,000/mm³.

had received a total dose of about 550 mg/m². There was a linear regression relationship between PEP/LVET ration and cumulative doses of 4'-epi-DOX. The comparative mean PEP/LVET ratio recorded after 550 mg/m² showed that the values were lower in patients given 4'-epi-DOX than in patients treated with DOX (Table 2). However, the difference was not significant.

THERAPEUTIC ACTIVITY

Table 3 shows the various types of tumor treated and their response to 4'-epi-DOX. Objective tumor regression was documented in a total of 33 of 99 patients evaluable for drug response after receiving doses of 50, 60, 75, and 90 mg/m². The total response rate was related to prior chemotherapy. In fact, in patients previously untreated objective tumor response oc-

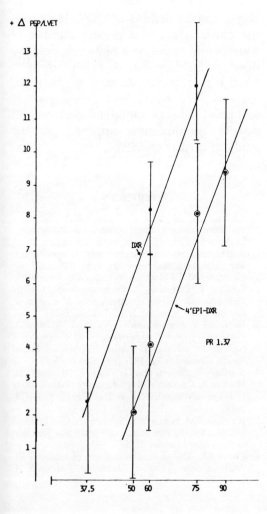

FIGURE 1. Variation of PEP-LVET ratio expressed as a percent change (+Δ%) from basal values, produced by different single doses of epi-DX in comparison with DX.

Table 2. Mean PEP/LVET Ratio After 500 mg/m^2 of Doxorubicin and 4'-Epidoxorubicin

	No. of Patients	Mean ± S.E.	t	p
Doxoru-bicin	23	0.416 ± 0.009		
4'-Epi-doxorubicin	14	0.401 ± 0.024	0.585	>0.05

colorectal cancer, which is another tumor unresponsive to DOX, for 26 and 14 weeks. In the remaining solid tumors the response duration ranged from a minimum of 8+ weeks to a maximum of 107+ weeks. In patients with hematologic malignancies both degree and duration of response could not be fully evaluated because, after receiving a few doses of 4'-epi-DOX, they were treated according to one of the conventional therapeutic programs.

Discussion

Results obtained during this clinical study showed that 4'-epi-DOX has some of the properties that, as pointed out by Carter,[6] could indicate its superiority to the parent compound and that are necessary to make a DOX analogue worthy of larger clinical trials.

In fact, just as in previously demonstrated experimental studies, 4'-epi-DOX showed reduced general and cardiac toxicity in comparison with DOX. In particular, gastrointestinal and hematologic toxicity were less severe than those seen at comparable doses of DOX and evaluation of acute and chronic cardiotoxicity, measured by systolic time intervals, showed a trend in favor of 4'-epi-DOX that produced lesser cardiac functional damage than DOX at comparable single and cumulative doses. Moreover, therapeutic results, also with the limits of present series, showed that 4'-epi-DOX could have a broader spectrum of activity than DOX with activity also in tumors considered resistant to DOX, such as melanoma and

curred in 49% compared with 20% for patients who had extensive previous drug therapy.

It is interesting to point out that complete remission of pulmonary metastases was observed in patients with two neoplasms, melanoma and renal cancer, which are known to be refractory to DOX. The remission duration lasted for 30 and 118 weeks, respectively. Partial response and objective improvement were also observed in two patients with metastatic

Table 3.   Therapeutic Activity of 4'-Epidoxorubicin in 99 Patients

Tumor Type	No. of Patients	Response[a]		
		CR	PR	OI
Melanoma	20	1	1	3
Breast cancer	13		3	4
Lung cancer	8			
Renal cancer	8	1	1	1
Head and neck cancer	5			1
Bladder cancer	5		1	
Colorectal cancer	6		1	1
Gastric cancer	1			
Hepatic cancer	1			
Ovarian cancer	2			
Endometrial cancer	2			
Testicular cancer	3			
Soft tissue sarcoma	6			
Osteosarcoma	1			
Thyroid cancer	2		1	
Kaposi's sarcoma	1		1	
Non-Hodgkin's lymphoma	9	2	4	2
Polycythemia vera	1	1		
Chronic lymphocytic leukemia	1		1	
Chronic myelogenous leukemia	2		2	
Primary site unknown	2			

[a]CR: complete remission; PR: partial response; OI: objective improvement.

renal cancer. From the point of view of the reduced general toxicity, the drug could be utilized with benefit in known combination regimens instead of DOX. However, the crucial goal, of a greater number of courses and therefore a higher cumulative dose of the drug can be safely administered before cardiac damage is observed, remains to be established. This important end point requires a more innovative, and possibly noninvasive, approach to the study of cardiac toxicity.

REFERENCES

1. Arcamone F, Di Marco A, Casazza AM: Chemistry and pharmacology of new antitumor anthracyclines. In *Advances Cancer Chemotherapy*. Umezawa, *et al.*, (Eds). Japan Science Society Press, Tokyo/University Park Press, Baltimore, 1978, pp 297–312.
2. Casazza AM, Di Marco A, Bertazzoli C, Formelli F, Giuliani F, Pratesi G: Antitumor activity, toxicity and pharmacological properties of 4'-epi-adriamycin. *Curr Chemother 2: 1257–1260, 1978.*
3. Bonfante V, Bonadonna G, Villani F, Martini A: Preliminary clinical experience with 4'-epi-doxorubicin in advanced human neoplasia. *Recent Results Cancer Res 74: 192–199, 1980.*
4. Bonfante V, Bonadonna G, Villani F, Di Fronzo G, Martini A, Casazza AM: Preliminary phase I study of 4'-epi-adriamycin. *Cancer Treat Rep 63: 915–918, 1979.*
5. Weissler AM, Harris WS, Schoenfeld CD: Bedside technics for the evaluation of ventricular function in man. *Am J Cardiol 23: 577–583, 1969.*
6. Carter SK: The clinical evaluation of analogs. III. Anthracyclines. *Cancer Chemother Pharmacol 4: 5–10, 1980.*

CHAPTER 24

Phase II Clinical Trial of 4'-Epidoxorubicin: An Interim Report

R. De Jager, P. Hurteloup, and G. Mathé

4'-Epidoxorubicin (4'-epi-DOX) is a stereoisomer of doxorubicin (DOX). The amino sugar daunosamine is replaced by its 4'-epi analogue (Fig. 1). 4'-Epi-DOX was selected for clinical trial on the basis of a higher therapeutic index than DOX in experimental tumor systems and lower cardiotoxicity in the rat and rabbit models.[1,2]

More recently, however, Dantchev et al.[3] showed that both compounds were equitoxic in the golden hamster cardiotoxicity model. Differences in drug distribution, metabolism, and excretion of 4'-epi-DOX and DOX have been reported in animals.[4]

Bonfante et al. reported the results of a phase I study in patients with advanced solid tumors given a single dose every 3 weeks. The pattern of toxicity of the two drugs appeared similar but 4'-epi-DOX appeared less toxic than DOX at the same doses. Myelosuppression was the major toxicity. This study did not define the maximal tolerated dose of 4'-epi-DOX and did not show that leukopenia was dose dependent following dose escalation up to 90 mg/m^2. However, since therapeutic activity similar to that of DOX was obtained with little toxicity with doses of 75–90 mg/m^2 of 4'-epi-DOX, it appeared that 4'-epi-DOX might have a higher therapeutic

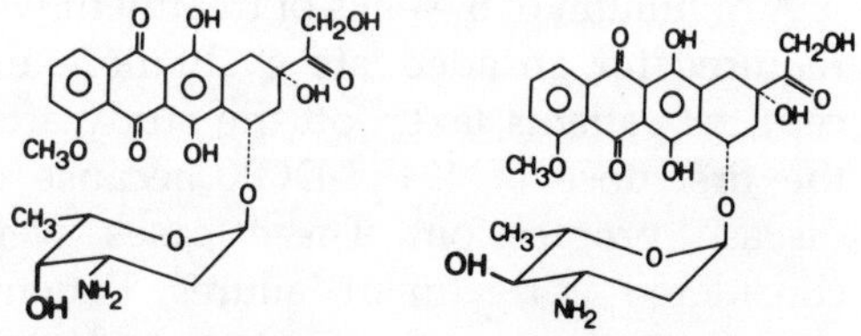

FIGURE 1. Chemical structure of doxorubicin (left) and 4'-epidoxorubicin (right).

index than DOX clinically as well.[5,6] On the basis of these results, the EORTC Clinical Screening Group initiated a broad clinical phase II study of 4'-epi-DOX in advanced solid tumors.

Materials and Methods

All patients entered in the study had histologically proven and progressive advanced solid tumors resistant to conventional treatment. The following criteria for eligibility were set: age 15–70 years, performance status: 0–3 (WHO), no prior radiation or chemotherapy within 3 weeks, white blood cell count (WBC) >3000/mm^3, platelet count >150,000/mm^3, normal hepatic and renal functions. Patients having received prior DOX treatment with a cumulative dose $\geq$250 mg/m^2 were not eligible for the study. Also excluded were patients with primary tumors or concurrent disease, such as uncontrolled infection, central nervous system metastases,

For the EORTC Clinical Screening Group, Institut de Cancérologie et d'Immunogénétique (INSERM U-50), Hôpital Paul-Brousse, Villejuif, France.

congestive heart failure, cardiac arrhythmia, bilateral bundle branch block, or a history of myocardial infarction.

All patients had measurable and/or evaluable lesions for response evaluation.

4'-epi-DOX was supplied by Farmitalia-Carlo Erba, Milan, Italy, as a red powder in 10 or 50-mg vials. Each dose of the drug was reconstituted with sterile water and administered as an intravenous bolus. 4'-epi-DOX, 75 mg/m^2, was given as a single I.V. dose repeated at 21-day intervals.

A minimum of 6 weeks of treatment was required for an adequate evaluation, except for patients taken off the study after the first dose of 4'-epi-DOX because of disease progression. These cases were considered as treatment failures. Patients showing a therapeutic response to 4'-epi-DOX had treatment discontinued when they reached a cumulative dose of 550 mg/m^2.

Therapeutic activity was evaluated according to WHO criteria.[7]

Minor regressions (<50% decrease in tumor size) were not taken into consideration. An objective response (complete [CR] or partial remission [PR]) required a minimum of 4 weeks from the time the tumor regression was first observed.

Results and Discussion

THERAPEUTIC ACTIVITY

At the time of this interim report (May 1981), 84 patients who had received 4'-epi-DOX 75 mg/m^2 I.V. every 3 weeks were available for treatment evaluation. Fifteen patients were not evaluable for therapeutic activity because of early death, protocol violation, or loss to follow-up. The distribution of treatment response by tumor type is given in Table 1.

A statistically significant number of patients, sufficient to detect therapeutic activity at the 20% level with 95% confidence interval, has been obtained only in breast cancer. The level of antitumor activ-

Table 1. 4'-Epidoxorubicin Phase II Trial. Therapeutic Activity

Diagnosis	No. of Patients	PR	No Change	Patient Died
Breast	22	6 (27%)	15	1
Head and Neck	11	0	11	—
Genito-urinary	6	0	6	—
Gastro-intestinal	5	0	2	3
Endometrium	5	1	3	1
Cervix	4	1	3	—
Ovary	3	—	3	—
Sarcoma	4	—	3	1
Bronchus	3	—	3	—
Melanoma	2	1	1	—
Skin epidermoid	2	1	1	—
Non-Hodgkin's lymphoma	2	1	1	—
Total	69			

ity observed in breast cancer (27%) is similar to what one would expect with DOX given as second-line treatment. Tumor regressions occurred in soft tissue disease (5 patients) and in pulmonary metastases (1 patient). In patients who did not receive prior DOX, 5 of 12 PR were obtained versus 1 of 10 PR in patients with prior DOX treatment. In this study there was no patient clinically resistant to DOX who achieved an objective remission with 4'-epi-DOX.

Therapeutic activity was also detected in single cases of endometrial carcinoma (liver and lung metastases), epidermoid carcinoma of the cervix (pulmonary metastases), melanoma (soft tissue disease), and non-Hodgkin's lymphoma (spleen).

Data are too scarce in the other tumor categories to exclude therapeutic activity at the present time.

TOXICITY

The analysis of toxicity was made on 79 patients according to the criteria of intolerance and toxicity (IT) used by the EORTC Clinical Screening Group (Table 2). The results are shown in Table 3.

Table 2. Codes for Evaluation of Toxicity and Efficacy

Evaluation of Intolerance and Toxicity (I.T.[a])

IT_0:   Absence of any evidence of toxicity.

IT_1:   Minor toxicity or toxicity easily countered by symptomatic treatment and/or not necessitating modification of the treatment.

IT_2:   Toxicity not responding adequately to symptomatic treatment and/or necessitating adaptation of the treatment (e.g., reduction and/or modification of dosage frequency) or delayed toxicity (occuring after the end of therapy).

IT_3:   Major toxicity necessitating discontinuation of the drug.

IT_4:   Toxicity having produced death.

IT_5:   Toxicity that could not be evaluated.

Evaluation of Efficacy

This is evaluated by taking into account the subjective, symptomatic and objective signs.

Subjective and Symptomatic Responses (S)

Only symptoms related to the treated malignant disease are to be taken in account:

S_0:   Aggravation, status quo or slight improvement

S_1:   Definite improvement

S_2:   Normalization of all symptoms

S_3:   Non-assessable effect

Objective Effect

The only effect (E) to be considered is that observed in lesions that can be assessed clinically or through x-rays at the end of the course of therapy, regardless of its duration.

E_0:   Aggravation

E_1:   Checking of progression of lesions or regression up to 20%

E_2:   Regression <50% in the volume of the tumor

E_3:   Regression >50% but incomplete

E_4:   Complete regression (normalization of all lesions)

[a] The abbreviation IT was adopted because it adedescribes the reactions observed and also because it avoids any confusion between the letter I and number 1, and also between the letter T (toxicity) and that used to represent tumoral extension in the TNM system.

At the dose of 75 mg/m², 4'-epi-DOX gave only minimal to moderate toxicity. No severe toxicity leading to discontinua-

Table 3. 4'-Epidoxorubicin: Phase II Trial, Toxicity

Type of Toxicity	Number of Patients (Total: 79)				
	IT_0	IT_1	IT_2	IT_3	IT_4
Nausea and vomiting	48	26	5	0	0
Stomatitis	77	2	0	0	0
Fever	48	22	9	0	0
Hair loss	43	28	0	0	0
Leukopenia	72	3	4	0	0
Thrombocytopenia	76	0	3	0	0
Cardiac	76	3	0	0	0
Renal or hepatic	79	0	0	0	0

tion of treatment (IT3) nor lethal toxicity (IT4) were encountered. Leukopenia and thrombocytopenia were seen in less than 10% of the patients. The most prevalent types of toxicity (IT1 + IT2) were nausea and/or vomiting and asthenia (occasionally with fever) recorded in a total of 40% of the patients. Hair loss was observed in approximately 65% of the cases and there was no renal or hepatic toxicity.

The cumulative dose distribution shows that the majority of patients received 300 mg/m² or less of 4'-epi-DOX. The highest cumulative dose reached was 600 mg/m² in two patients. There was no case of congestive heart failure; 3 cases of acute reversible electrocardiographic (ECG) abnormalities were recorded, consisting of tachyarrhythmias with S-T wave alteration (in one patient who had received a cumulative dose of 225 mg/m²) and two cases of decrease in the voltage of the QRS complex, including one in a patient who had received prior DOX treatment (cumulative DOX dose <250 mg/m²). Cardiotoxicity was not the reason for 4'-epi-DOX treatment interruption in any case.

Conclusion

Treatment with 4'-epi-DOX has resulted in objective tumor regressions in several types of solid tumors. The therapeutic activity against breast cancer is similar to that of DOX used as second-line treatment, confirming the results obtained by other investigators. The fact that these responses were obtained with 4'-epi-DOX at a dose level (75 mg/m²) resulting in only minimal to moderate toxicity may reflect the fact that 4'-epi-DOX has a better therapeutic index than DOX. However, the study design of this single arm phase II clinical trial does not allow us to draw such a conclusion. To test this hypothesis, a straightforward prospective randomized study comparing 4'-epi-DOX to DOX is needed. Furthermore, since therapeutic activity may be dose dependent, it appears desirable also to evaluate the therapeutic activity of 4'-epi-DOX at higher doses. Besides attempting to demonstrate that 4'-epi-DOX is at least as active but less toxic than DOX, a better comparison of the two drugs in terms of therapeutic activity should be obtained by testing them at equitoxic doses.

In addition to comparing the therapeutic indices of the two drugs in DOX-sensitive tumors (i.e., breast cancer), it is necessary to test the antitumor activity of 4'-epi-DOX against the full spectrum of tumors in disease-oriented phase II studies. The activity of 4'-epi-DOX in melanoma detected in this study and in the study by Bonfante et al.[6] suggests that the spectrum of activity of the two drugs may not overlap entirely.

The risk of cardiotoxicity cannot be evaluated from this multicentric clinical trial because of the arbitrary cut off cumulative dose of 550 mg/m² of 4'-epi-DOX and because monitoring consisted only of ECG tracings in the majority of cases. However, because more patients will receive higher cumulative doses of 4'-epi-DOX with or without prior DOX, one should stress the importance of careful monitoring of the cardiac function by echography or radionuclide angiography in order to document early cardiotoxicity.

The preliminary results of this early phase II trial of 4'-epi-DOX suggest that the drug may have a broad spectrum of activity against solid tumors. The therapeutic index of 4'-epi-DOX compared to that of DOX and the clinical cross-resistance between the two drugs remain open questions to be investigated in future clinical trials.

NOTE

The EORTC Clinical Screen Group:

Chairman: P. Cappelaere; Secretary: G. Mathé; Trial Coordinator: P. Hurteloup.

Members — *Bordeaux:* M. Caudry, J. Chauvergne; Montpellier: J. Gary-Bobo, B. Serrou; Nice: M. Namer, M. Schneider; Strasbourg: R. Keiling, T. Klein, J.M. Lang; Lille: P. Cappelaere; *Villejuif (ICIG):* G. Mathé, J.L. Misset, F. de Vassal, M. Hayat; *Villejuif (IGR):* J. Rouesse, G. Brulé, F. May-Levin; Bescançon: S. Schraub, P. Hurteloup; *Toulouse:* J.P. Armand; Grenoble: R. Shaerer; *Rouen:* P. Bastit, H. Piquet, C. Jeanne; *Reims:* S. Nasca, A. Cattan, Ch. Pourny; *Coimbra (Portugal):* C. de Oliveira; *Dijon:* J. Guerrin, P. Fargeot; *Saint-Cloud:* B. Clavel, J. Berlié; Lyon: F. Cheix, E. Pommatau, N. Bonnafous; Saint-Etienne: P. Serpentié; *Granada (Spain):* M. Delgado; Nantes: O. Godin; *Brussels (Belgium):* C. Cauchie, R. Maurus; *Rotterdam (Holland):* T.J. Kuipers.

REFERENCES

1. Casazza AM, Di Marco A, Bertazzoli C, Formelli F, Giuliani F, Pratesi G. Anti-tumor activity, toxicity and pharmacological properties of 4'-epi-adriamycin. *Current Chemother* 2: 1257–1260, 1978.
2. Casazza AM, Di Marco A, Bonadonna G, Bonfante V, Bertazzoli C, Bellini O, Pratesi G, Sala L, Ballerini L: Effects of modifications in position 4 of the chromophore or in position 4' of the aminosugar, on the antitumor activity and toxicity of daunorubicin and doxorubicin. In *Anthracyclines: Current Status and New Developments*, Crooke ST, Reich ST (Eds). Academic Press, New York, 1980, pp 403–439.
3. Dantchev D, Paintrand M, Bourut C, Pignot I, Maral R, Mathé G: Comparative experimental study and evaluation of the degree of cardiotoxicity and alopecia of twelve different anthracyclins using the golden hamster model. In *Anthracyclines*, Mathé G, De Jager R, Maral R (Eds). Masson Publishing USA, New York, 1983.
4. Broggini M, Colombo T, Martini A, Donelli MG: Studies on the comparative distribution and

biliary excretion of doxorubicin and 4'-epi-doxo-rubicin in mice and rats. *Cancer Treat Rep 64: 897–904, 1980.*

5. Bonfante V, Bonadonna G, Villani F, Di Fronzo G, Martini A, Casazza AM: Preliminary phase I-study of 4'-epi-adriamycin. *Cancer Treat Rep 63: 915–918, 1979.*

6. Bonfante V, Bonadonna G, Villani F, Martini A: Prelminiary clinical experience with 4'-epi-doxo-rubicin in advanced human neoplasia. *Recent Results Cancer Res 74: 192–199, 1980.*

7. *W.H.O. Handbook for Reporting Results of Cancer Treatment.* WHO Offset Publication, no. 48, Geneva, 1979.

CHAPTER 25

Rubidazone

Cl. Jacquillat, M. Weil, M. F. Auclerc, J. Maral, and J. Bernard

The experimental activity of this semi-synthetic derivative was described in 1972 by Maral et al.[1] It is less cytotoxic *in vitro* than daunorubicin or doxorubicin. Autoradiographs of KB cells showed that inhibition of precursor incorporation was more progressive and lasted for a longer time with rubidazone than with daunorubicin or doxorubicin.

In L1210 cells Bachur showed that cellular incorporation occurred by active transport and that there was a close correlation between inhibition and cellular accumulation that varied with rubidazone, daunorubicin, and doxorubicin.

Rubidazone is less toxic in mice (DL_{150}, S.C., I.P., or I.V.) and better tolerated in dogs and rabbits at doses from 0.25 to 0.75 mg/kg I.V. for a long period. However, it is cardiotoxic in rats[2,3] and in hamsters.[4] In rabbits rubidazone is less toxic than daunorubicin or adriamycin. The therapeutic index of rubidazone, daunorubicin and doxorubicin are close to each other on sarcoma 180 and L1210 leukemia.[1,5] In experimental tumors there is a cross-resistance between rubidazone, daunorubicin, and adriamycin.[6] Pharmacokinetic study of rubidazone showed that the first metabolite that appeared during infusion was daunorubicin. However, the amount of daunorubicinol is decreased during the first 12 hours, suggesting the inhibition of daunorubicin reductase.[7]

Thus, rubidazone may be considered as a prodrug of daunorubicin with specific kinetic parameters. Experimentally, this drug is less toxic, less cardiotoxic, and as active as daunorubicin: its metabolism is different from the other anthracyclines.

Clinical Activity

ACTIVITY OF RUBIDAZONE IN MONOCHEMOTHERAPY

As shown in Table 1, we treated 299 patients by rubidazone alone for various malignancies, mainly acute leukemias. In the first 56 patients the median necessary dose to achieve complete remission (CR) has been 23 mg/kg. A course of 4 mg/kg/day for 5 days was given initially and the additional doses have been given intermittently according to bone marrow aspiration picture. In these patients, many of whom had advanced relapses, the rate of CR was 45%.

As shown in Table 2, these encouraging results were confirmed in 1976, since the rate of CR in 40 patients with advanced acute lymphocytic leukemia (ALL) was 55%.

In 107 patients with acute myelogenous leukemia (AML), the global rate of CR was 53%, and in first attacks it was 57% (Table 3). Thus in the following varieties of AML (M1, M2, M4, M6), rubidazone is as active and better tolerated than daunorubicin.

But the main indication of rubidazone in acute granulocytic leukemias is the monoblastic variety (M5). Patients with this disease have high blastic counts (median value

Service d'Oncologie Médicale, Hopital de la Salpetrière, Service du Prof. Jacquillat, Paris Cedex 13, France

159

Table 1. Results of 299 Patients Treated in Phase I or II with Rubidazone Alone

Published Results (Year of Publication)	ALL	AML	Acute Monocytic Leukemia	Acute Promyelocytic Leukemia	Acute CML	Non-Hodgkin's Lymphoma	Solid Tumors	Total
1971	24	32						56
1976	44	107		1		4		156
1980			57					57
Non-Published Results					9		21	30
Total	68	139	57	1	9	4	21	299

60,000 per mm³), bulky tumoral infiltration, and often gum and skin involvement.

Muramidase is high in plasma and urine and its values are correlated with blastic cell counts as well as with blood urea nitrogen and creatinine increase in blood and with biological symptoms of disseminated intravascular coagulation (fall of V factor, fall of fibrin, increase of fibrinogen degradation products). Drastic cellular lysis impairs renal failure; thus, out of 30 patients treated with daunorubicin, 11 patients died with symptoms of renal failure. As shown on Table 4, the rate of CR with rubidazone is 73% which is a significant improvement compared to that of daunorubicin. Combination of rubidazone with

Aracytine or Aracytine and Vehem are presently one progress in this disease.

By contrast, in acute promyelocytic leukemias and in leukemias with a short doubling time and clinical symptoms of hypoxia, rapid activity is necessary and daunorubicin seems to be more indicated than rubidazone.

In 9 patients with chronic myelogenous leukemia (CML) in the acute phase, two short CR were observed. In 4 patients with non-Hodgkin's lymphomas a short CR was observed in a patient with the lymphoblastic variety and a more lasting one in a patient with the diffuse large cell variety. In 21 patients with solid tumors (16 epidermoid tongue epitheliomas, three meta-

Table 2. Results in 40 Patients with ALL

	Initial Resistance	First Relapse	Second Relapse	Third Relapse	Total
CR	4	7	8	3	22
PR		1	2		3
Failures		2	6	4	12
Induction death	1	1		1	3
Total	5	11	16	8	40

Table 3. Results in 107 Patients Treated with Rubidazone in Acute Myelogenous Leukemia

	First Attack without TT	First Attack with TT	First Relapse	Second Relapse	Total
CR	40 (57%)	2	13 (50%)	1	56 (53%)
PR	3	1			4
Resistance	12	2	9	2	25
Induction death	15	1	4	2	22
Total	70	6	26	5	107

Table 4. Induction Results in Acute Monocytic Leukemia (M5) with Rubidazone

	CR	PR	Fail-ures	Induc-tion Death	Total
Before 1970	8 (19%)	2	18	14	42
Dauno-rubicin or combina-tion with dauno-rubicin	12 (40%)	2	5	11	30
Rubidazone	42 (73%)	1	5	9	57
Combina-tion with Rubidazone	7 (87%)			1	8

Table 5. Posology of Protocol 10 LAL 76—Paris

Score 1	Score 2	Score 3	Score 4 (Patients ≥50 Years)	Drugs[a]
1,5	2	2,25	2	VCR (mg/m^2), day #1
400	500	600	500	Ctx (mg/m^2), day #1
20 × 3	30 × 3	40 × 3	30 × 3	DNR (mg/m^2), days 1, 2, 3
40 × 3	60 × 3	80 × 3	60 × 3	BHDNR (mg/m^2), days 1, 2, 3
40	60	80	60	Prednisone (mg/m^2/d) until CR
40 × 3	60 × 3	80 × 3	60 × 3	Ara-C (mg/m^2) days 1, 2, 3 cont. perf.

Levamisole: 150 mg/m^2/day for 3 days every 2 weeks for induction and remission

[a]VCR: vincristine; Ctx: cyclophosphamide; DNR: daunorubicin; BHDNR: Rubidazone.

static breast, one kidney, and one rhabdomyosarcoma) one partial regression (PR) was observed (metastatic breast).

COMBINATIONS WITH RUBIDAZONE

Since 1976, within the framework of the French Cooperative Group of the Hematology Society, several phase III studies using Rubidazone in combination with other drugs were activated.

In ALL we compared rubidazone and daunorubicin in a combination including prednisone, vincristine, and cyclophosphamide with or without cytosine arabinoside (Ara-C). As shown on Table 5, the doses varied according to the prognostic score.

In children induction results are the same with rubidazone and with daunorubicin (Table 6). In adults, by contrast, results are significantly better with rubidazone. Out of 17 patients who died during induction, only one was treated by rubidazone. In children the duration of CR is lenghtened by Ara-C. In adults, Ara-C is additive in the daunorubicin arm but not in the rubidazone arm. In adults the rate of CR at 2 years is 35% for Ara-C and rubidazone, 40% for rubidazone, 28% for Ara-C and daunorubicin and 18% for daunorubicin.

In AML, rubidazone and Ara-C were combined in several protocols. Induction results indicate that more CR are achieved when anthracycline doses are increased. Duration of CR remains short with a median at 12 months but 25% of the patients remain disease-free at 4 years.

TOXICITY

Rubidazone is generally well tolerated. In some patients allergic reactions may occur and increase of histamine in blood was recognized with rubidazone as with other anthracyclines.

In leukemias, aplasias preceding CR are always observed. They appear around day 5 and last for about 15 days. In solid tumors, hematologic toxicity may appear for doses exceeding 120 mg/m².

Table 6. Results of Combination with Rubidazone in Children with ALL

	Prednisone Vincristine Cyclophosphamide Daunorubicin	Prednisone Vincristine Cyclophosphamide Rubidazone	Prednisone Vincristine Cyclophosphamide Daunorubicin Ara-C	Prednisone Vincristine Cyclophosphamide Rubidazone Ara-C	Total
CR	51 (86.5%)	54 (87%)	52 (92.8%)	54 (90%)	211 (91%)
PR	1	2		1	4
Resistance	3	4		3	10
Induction death	4	2	4	2	12
Total	59	62	56	60	237

Experimental studies demonstrate that rubidazone is cardiotoxic but to a lesser degree than daunorubicin or doxorubicin. This has been confirmed in patients. Except in two cases with cardiac history were repolarization disturbances led to early drug withdrawal, no clinical cardiac toxicity was observed during first attacks after mean doses of 1000 mg/m². But the same doses led to cardiac failures when they are given after daunorubicin (500 mg/m²) or when they were followed during further relapses by additional courses of rubidazone (1000 mg/m²) or daunorubicin (400 mg/m²) or even m-AMSA (1000 mg/m²).

We conclude that rubidazone is as active and less toxic than daunorubicin in most cases of acute leukemia. In contrast to daunorubicin it may be given intermittently. It is the best present treatment for AML. It is clearly better tolerated than daunorubicin in adult cases of ALL. As with daunorubicin, it is less active than doxorubicin or diethoxyacetoxy daunorubicin in solid tumors.

ACKNOWLEDGMENTS

This work was supported by INSERM Contract, Commission 8 (Prof. Laudat); Franco-American Committee for Research on Cancer (INSERM); Unit 232, INSERM; and USPHS Research Grant, CA 13 239-05 of the National Cancer Institute.

REFERENCES

1. Maral R, Ponsinet G, Jolles G: Etude de l'activité anti-tumorale expérimentale d'un nouvel antibiotique semi-synthétique: la Rubidazone (22 050 RP). C R Acad Sci [D] (Paris) 275 (2): 301-304, 1972.
2. Zbinden G, Braendle, E: Toxicologic screening of daunorubicin (NSC 82151), adriamycin (NSV 123127), and their derivatives in rats. Cancer Chemother Rep 59: (4), 707-715, 1975.
3. Bachmann E, Weber E, Zbinden G: Effects of seven anthracycline antibiotics on electrocardiogram and mitochondrial function of rat hearts. Agents Actions 5(4): 383-393, 1975.
4. Dnchev D, Slioussartchouk V, Paintrand M, Bourut C, Hayat M, Mathé, G: Etude ultrastructurale de la cardiotoxicité et des alterations de la peau chez le hamster doré après traitement avec huit différentes anthracyclines. Soc Biol (Paris) 173 (2): 393-413, 1979.
5. Daalen Wetters T Van, Alberts DS, Wood DA: Rubidazone (R) versus adriamycin (A): Studies of their efficacy ratios (E.R.) in the spleen colony assay (SCA) system. Proc Am Assoc Cancer Res 17: 67, 1976.
6. Johnson RK, Ovejera AA, Goldin A: Activity of anthracyclines against an adriamycin (NSC (12311127). Resistant subline of P388 leukemia with special emphasis on cinerubin A (NSC 18334) Cancer Treat Rep 60 (1): 99-102, 1976.
7. Baurain R, Deprez-de Campeneere D, Trouet A: Distribution and metabolism of rubidazone and daunorubicin in mice. Cancer Chemother Pharmacol 1979, 2 (1): 37-41, 1979.

CHAPTER 26

Experimental and Clinical Data on Pharmacokinetics and Efficacy of the Daunorubicin-DNA and Adriamycin-DNA Complexes

R. Hulhoven

This chapter summarizes the data available on experimental and clinical use of the daunorubicin (DNR)- and Adriamycin (ADM)-DNA complexes.

Experimental Data

The DNR-DNA and ADM-DNA complexes have been proposed as lysosomotropic agents for cancer chemotherapy. This hypothesis was based on *in vitro* experiments performed in several tumor cell lines. The first results obtained in DBA/2 mice bearing L1210 leukemia showed a better therapeutic efficacy and a lower toxicity of these complexes, particularly in the case of the ADM-DNA complex.[1,2] However, other investigators using L1210 leukemia from another origin or transplanted in other mice species, or solid tumors, were unable to show any therapeutic advantage of this complex.[3] Acute cardiotoxic effect appeared reduced when these complexes were infused in isolated hearts.[4] Experimental pharmacokinetics of these complexes were studied in mice[5,6] and rabbits,[7,8] this last species being more suitable because of the possibility of infusion (large viscous volume!), of repeated blood sampling and of investigation of car-

Laboratory of Pharmacotherapy (Prof. C. Harvengt), Catholic University of Louvain, Brussels, Belgium

diovascular toxicity. Furthermore, metabolism of anthracyclines in this species is more similar to human beings than are rats or mice.[9] In addition, experiments conducted with these complexes *in vitro* did not confirm the lysosomotropic theory.[10-12]

We have studied the pharmacokinetics of the DNR-DNA complex in conscious rabbits using an original high pressure liquid chromatography (HPLC) method[13] and ^{125}I-DNA. The injection of a 5-mg dose of complexed DNR induced acute hypervolemic cardiac failure in two of five rabbits.[7] Therefore this mode of administration was discarded and a 4-hour infusion period was chosen. During this infusion period, the plasma levels of DNR and DNA progressively increased. The dissociation of the complex in the bloodstream occurred quickly, 80% of DNR leaving the carrier during the infusion.[8] This was also observed in one rabbit injected with 2.5 mg/kg of the labeled complex. These results were confirmed by others in mice, using injection of a large dose of this complex, this animal species tolerating better hypervolemia. In this model, the dissociation of the ADM-DNA complex appeared somewhat less pronounced.[6] It must be pointed out that the reticuloendothelial system (R.E.S.) blockade induced by colloidal carbon injections did not modify the DNR plasma kinetics.[14] The study of tissue distribution in rabbits exhibited a marked reduction of DNR levels in heart and lungs when DNR was infused over 4 hours instead of bolus injected. A slight reduction of DNR uptake in these tissues was observed after infusion of the DNR-DNA complex when compared with the free drug infused under the same conditions. Similar experiments performed with these complexes in a few rats showed a slightly reduced uptake of DNR-DNA and ADM-DNA complexes in the heart toward the free drugs.[15] Data about chronic cardiac toxicity in animals treated with these complexes are not available, so far.

Clinical Data

The efficacy of the DNA complexes has been established in human patients, in phase I and II trials.[16-21] Some phase III trials have been conducted. Preliminary results of four randomized studies have been published.[22,23] Three of these studies were performed in our department of hematology, the final results of which are summarized below:

1. A trial in childhood acute lymphocytic leukemia(ALL), with 64 patients, compared two polychemotherapy protocols, the first one including DNR-DNA, and the second one, ADM-DNA. There was a slight, but not statistically significant, advantage in favor of the second arm, in the case of poor prognosis ALL.
2. A trial in acute myelogenous leukemia (AML), with 90 patients, compared the association of DNR and Ara-C or DNR-DNA and Ara-C. No statistically significant difference could be observed between the two arms concerning efficacy or toxicity.
3. A trial in anaplastic bronchial carcinoma, with 54 patients, compared the efficacy of ADM or ADM-DNA. There was a slight, but not statistically significant, advantage in favor of the uncomplexed drug.

A further trial comparing both drugs in polychemotherapy protocol is still in progress. As yet, no difference is observed between the two arms of this protocol.

WHAT ABOUT PHARMACOKINETICS OF THESE COMPLEXES IN HUMANS?

Pharmacokinetics of the DNR-DNA complex in leukemic patients were very similar to the ones observed in rabbits,[24] a fivefold higher DNR plasma level being achieved at the end of the complex infusion. The difference toward free drug infusion was not more significant after 4 hours. Incomplete data from others confirmed this trend.[25] Preliminary pharmacokinetic comparisons of the infusion of ADM versus the infusion of the ADM-DNA complex showed similar ADM plasma profiles.[26,27]

WHAT ABOUT CARDIOTOXICITY OF THESE COMPLEXES?

Patients receiving cumulative doses as high as 1500 mg/m^2 of the complexed anthracyclines showed no clinical evidence of cardiac failure. However, in a few patients, investigated by endomyocardial biopsy, myocardial tissue damage, not very different from that seen after the free drugs, was observed.[28] Furthermore, it has been reported that changing the sequence or the mode of administration of anthracyclines can induce less cardiotoxicity.[29,30]

Conclusion

Experimental and clinical pharmacokinetic studies demonstrated the quick dissociation of these complexes. No therapeutic advantage versus the free drugs were observed so far. Perhaps somewhat less cardiotoxicity could be achieved, but sensitive methods are needed in order to substantiate this particular point.

ACKNOWLEDGMENTS

Dr. N. Fauconnier-Dehasque and Dr. A. Bosly are sincerely acknowledged for their collaboration in the collection of the clinical data. Thanks are due to Dr. J. Binon for the statistical analyses and to Miss M. P. Berckmans for typing this manuscript.

REFERENCES

1. Trouet A, Deprez-Decampeneere D, de Duve C: Chemotherapy through lysosomes with a DNA-daunorubicin complex. *Nature [New Biol]* 239: 110–112, 1972.
2. Trouet A, Deprez-Decampeneere D, Desmedt-Malengreaux M, Atassi G: Experimental leukemia chemotherapy with a lysosomotropic adriamycin-DNA complex. *Eur J Cancer* 10: 405–411, 1974.
3. Atassi G, Tagnon HJ, Staquet M: Comparison of adriamycin and adriamycin-DNA complex in chemotherapy of experimental tumors and metastases. In *Adriamycin Review*, European Press:Medikon, Ghent, Belgium, 1975, pp 62–69.
4. Langslet A, Øye I, Lie SO: Decreased cardiac toxicity of adriamycin and daunorubicin when bound to DNA. *Acta Pharmacol Toxicol [Copenh]* 35: 379–385, 1974.
5. Ohnuma T, Holland JF, Chen JH: Pharmacological and therapeutic efficacy of daunomycin-DNA complex in mice. *Cancer Res* 35: 1767–1772, 1975.
6. Deprez-Decampeneere D, Baurain R, Huybrechts M, Trouet A: Comparative study of the toxicity, pharmacology and therapeutic activity of daunorubicin-DNA and doxorubicin-DNA complexes. *Cancer Chemother Pharmacol* 2: 25–30, 1979.
7. Hulhoven R, Desager JP, Sokal G, Harvengt C: Plasma levels and biotransformation of infused daunorubicin and daunorubicin-DNA complex in rabbits — a preliminary report. *Eur J Cancer* 13: 1065–1069, 1977.
8. Hulhoven R: Daunorubicin, daunorubicinol and DNA plasma kinetics after i.v. administration of daunorubicin-DNA complex in the rabbit. *Biomedicine* 29: 164–167, 1978.
9. Felsted RL, Bachur NR: Mammalian carbonyl-reductase. *Drug Metab Rev* 11: 1–60, 1980.
10. Seeber S, Brucksch KP, Seeber B, Schmidt CG: Cytostatic efficacy of DNA complexes of adriamycin, daunomycin and actinomycin-D. (I) Comparative studies in Novikoff hepatoma, human mammary carcinoma cells and human leukemic leukocytes. *Z Krebsforsch* 89: 75–86, 1977.
11. Skovsgaard T: In vitro and in vivo study of cross resistance between daunorubicin and daunorubicin-DNA complex in Ehrlich ascites tumor. *Cancer Chemother Pharmacol* 2: 43–47, 1979.
12. Zenebergh A, Schneider YJ, Trouet A: Comparative studies of the accumulation of doxorubicin and doxorubicin-DNA in various cell lines. *Biochem Pharmacol* 29: 1035–1040, 1980.
13. Hulhoven R, Desager JP: Quantitative determination of low levels of Daunomycin and daunomycinol in plasma by high-performance liquid chromatography. *J Chromatogr* 125: 369–374, 1976
14. Hulhoven R, Harvengt C: Daunorubicin, daunorubicinol and DNA plasma kinetics after i.v. administration of daunorubicin-DNA complex in the rabbit. II — Effects of R.E.S.-blockade. *Biomedicine* 33: 44–47, 1980.
15. Blanchard JC, Schneider YJ, Baurain R, Trouet A: Accumulation, metabolism and subcellular localizations of daunorubicin, doxorubicin and their DNA-complexes in rat heart ventricules. *Eur J Cancer* 17: 297–305, 1981.
16. Sokal G, Trouet A, Michaux JL, Cornu G: Daunorubicin-DNA complex : Preliminary trials in human leukemia. *Eur J Cancer* 9: 391–392, 1973.
17. Cornu G, Michaux JL, Sokal G, Trouet A: Daunorubicin-DNA : Further clinical trials in acute non lymphoblastic leukemia. *Eur J Cancer* 10: 695–700, 1974.
18. Longueville J, Maisin H: Combined therapy with adriamycin-DNA, vincristine and medroxy-progesterone acetate in metastatic breast cancer. In: *Adriamycin Review*, European Press: Medikon, Ghent, Belgium, 1975, pp 260–267.
19. Lie SO, Lie KK, Glomstein A: Clinical and pharmacologic studies with adriamycin-DNA complex in children with malignant disease. *Cancer Chemother Pharmacol* 2: 61–66. 1979.
20. Benjamin RS, Burgess MA, Bodey GP, McCredie DB, Freireich EJ: A phase I-II study of adriamycin-DNA complex. *Proc Am Assoc Cancer Res* 18: 305, 1977.
21. Rozencweig M, Kenis Y, Atassi G, Staquet M, Durarte-Karim M: DNA-Adriamycin complex : Preliminary results in animals and man. *Cancer Chemother Rep* 6: 131–136, 1975.
22. Ferrant A, Hulhoven R, Bosly A, Cornu G, Michaux JL, Sokal G: Clinical trials with daunorubicin-DNA and adriamycin-DNA in acute lymphoblastic leukemia of childhood, acute non lymphoblastic leukemia, and bronchogenic carcinoma. *Cancer Chermother Pharmacol* 2: 67–71, 1979.
23. Gahrton G, Björkholm M, Breuning G, Christenson I, Engstedt L, Franzen S, et al: Treatment of acute non lymphoblastic leukemia in adults with daunorubicin-DNA complex — a preliminary report. *Cancer Chermother Pharmacol* 2: 73–76, 1979.
24. Hulhoven R, Sokal G, Harvengt C: Human pharmacokinetics of the daunorubicin-DNA complex. An alternative view of the lysosomotropic theory. *Cancer Chemother Pharmacol* 3: 243–247, 1979.
25. Andersson B, Andersson I, Beran M, Ehrsson H, Eksborg S: Liquid chromatography monitoring of daunorubicin and daunorubicinol in plasma from leukemic patients treated with daunorubicin or the daunorubicin-DNA complex. *Cancer Chemother Pharmacol* 2: 15–17, 1979.
26. Staquet M, Rozencweig M, Duarte-Karim M, Kenis Y: Pharmacokinetics of adriamycin and adriamycin-DNA complex in mice and man. *Eur J Cancer* 13: 433–435, 1977.

27. Kummen M, Lie KK, Lie SO: A pharmacokinetic evaluation of free and DNA complexed adriamycin: A preliminary study in children with malignant disease. *Acta Pharmacol Toxicol 42: 212–218, 1978.*

28. Benjamin RS, Mason JW, Billingham ME: Cardiac toxicity of adriamycin-DNA complex and Rubidazone — evaluation by ECG and endomyocardial biopsy. *Cancer Treat Rep 62: 935–939, 1978.*

29. Weiss AJ, Metter GE, Fletcher WS, Wilson WL, Grage TB, Ramirez G: Studies on adriamycin using a weekly regimen demonstrating its clinical effectiveness and lack of cardiotoxicity. *Cancer Treat Rep 60: 813–822, 1976.*

30. Praga C, Beretta G, Vigo PL, Lenaz GR, Pollini C, Bonadonna G, *et al.*: Adriamycin cardiotoxicity —a survey of 1273 patients. *Cancer Treat Rep, 63: 827–834, 1979.*

CHAPTER 27

Carminomycin — A Detailed Toxicity Study

M. M. de Planque, G. P. C. Simonetti, W. W. ten Bokkel Huinink, and J. G. McVie

Carminomycin is a new anthracycline antitumor antibiotic isolated from the mycelia of *Actinomadura carminata*. Carminomycin is stereochemically similar to daunorubicin. The molecule differs from daunorubicin in that the aglycone is a desmethyldaunorubicin. Biochemically it is closely related to doxorubicin.[1]

Initial studies in the USSR showed antitumor activity in a variety of animal tumor systems including L1210 and sarcoma 180. Toxicity was studied in a variety of animal models and appeared to be predominantly hematological and gastrointestinal. Cardiac toxicity was studied employing the Zbinden rat model and the acute cardiac toxicity model of Merski and both studies revealed less cardiac damage than observed with doxorubicin.[2,3]

Both Russian and American studies have shown carminomycin to be orally absorbed. Toxicity studies in mice revealed a ratio of the LD_{50} of oral to intravenous administration of 2:1. In man at a dose of 36 mg/m^2 free carminomycin was detected in the plasma.[1,4]

Clinical data from Russian studies indicated a spectrum of antitumor activity comparable to that of doxorubicin. Two dose schedules were employed predominantly in these studies: 7.5 mg/m^2 twice weekly for three weeks, repeated every 4 weeks, and 5.5 mg/m^2 daily × 5, repeated every three weeks, resulting in a total dose of 45 mg/m^2 and 27.5 mg/m^2 per course. Toxicity compared to that of doxorubicin was found to be less, consisting of nausea and vomiting, mild leukopenia and thrombocytopenia, and some alopecia. No cardiomyopathy was reported. In the United States clinical data were published concerning 17 cancer patients treated with escalating doses of 1–15 mg/m^2 I.V. carminomycin. Mild myelotoxicity occurred at doses of 15 mg/m^2 administered every 4 weeks. No therapeutic effects were noted, but these doses were well below the clinically effective doses employed in the Russian studies.[5]

Material and Methods

From August 1980–October 1981 nine white female patients, one with advanced soft tissue sarcoma and eight with advanced breast carcinoma, received carminomycin during EORTC phase II clinical trials.[6,7] Patients resistant to carminomycin were crossed over to doxorubicin. Patients were eligible when they had progressive residual or metastatic soft tissue sarcoma or advanced breast carcinoma. They were required to have no evidence of limited bone marrow reserve, renal or severe hepatic dysfunction, congestive heart failure or ECG abnormalities. Performance status according to Karnofsky had to be equal to or above 50.

Clinical Research Unit, Dept. of Internal Medicine, Antoni van Leeuwenhoekhuis, Netherlands Cancer Institute, Amsterdam, the Netherlands.

Pretreatment clinical examination included history, tumor measurements, complete blood count, renal and liver function studies, electrolytes, appropriate x-ray studies, including chest x-ray, bone scan, ECG, and ejection fraction measurement by gated equilibrium blood pool scintigraphy. Complete blood counts and chemistry were repeated at least weekly. Cardiac evaluation by ECG and ejection fraction was repeated prior to and 24 hours after each carminomycin administration.

Patients were seen weekly for clinical evaluation and assessment of Karnofsky performance status and WHO toxicity grading.[8] Radiologic or scintigraphic studies were performed when indicated. Patient data are summarized in Table 1. Most breast cancer patients had prior radiotherapy, hormone exposure and non-anthracycline chemotherapy.

Three patients had abnormal liver function studies. Patients 5 and 6 had elevated alkaline phosphatase, γGT and 5-nucleotidase, patient 6 had also mildly elevated SGOT and SGPT. Patient 7 had only a slightly elevated γGT. Bilirubin was normal in all three patients. These values were unaltered throughout the course of carminomycin therapy. No other patients showed abnormal liver function tests before or after therapy.

Carminomycin was administered by rapid intravenous injection every 3 weeks.

Drug administration was postponed by 1 week if there was no hematologic recovery (WBC > 3.0 × 10⁹/L, platelets > 100 × 10⁹/L) from the previous course at the scheduled treatment time.

Pharmacokinetic analysis of carminomycin and carminomycinol in plasma of every patient was carried out for 7 days after the first course. These results are reported by Lankelma et al.[9]

Results

Eight breast cancer patients started carminomycin therapy at a dose of 18 mg/m². One soft tissue sarcoma patient received carminomycin at an initial dose of 20 mg/m².

They received 1-3 doses of carminomycin resulting in a total of 21 courses evaluable for toxicity. Seven patients continued therapy after the first course, but most of them had to have the dosages adjusted due to hematological toxicity, predominantly leukopenia. Two patients had their second course postponed to day 29 and 34 before there was hematological recovery. Only four patients had platelet counts below 100 × 10⁹/L none below 30 × 10⁹/L. Hematological side effects of the first course are summarized in Figures 1–3.

Except for hematological toxicity no major side effects were encountered. No nausea and vomiting occurred, only some

Table 1. Patient Characteristics

Patient	Age	Diagnosis	Prior Radio/Chemotherapy	Metastases
1	57 yrs	Abdominal soft tissue Sarcoma (fibrosarcoma)	—	—
			—	—
2	37 yrs	Breast carcinoma R	CMF[a]	S/V
3	60 yrs	Breast carcinoma L	XRT/CMF	S/V
4	68 yrs	Breast carcinoma R	XRT/CMF	S
5	64 yrs	Breast carcinoma L	XRT/CMF	S/B/V
6	35 yrs	Breast carcinoma R	XRT/CMF	S/B/V
7	57 yrs	Breast carcinoma R	XRT/CMF	S/B/V
8	35 yrs	Breast carcinoma L	XRT/CMF	S
9	69 yrs	Breast carcinoma R	XRT/CMF	S/B/V

[a]CMF: cyclophosphamide, methotrexate, 5-fluorouracil; XRT: radiotherapy; S: skin, soft tissue; B: bone, V: visceral metastases.

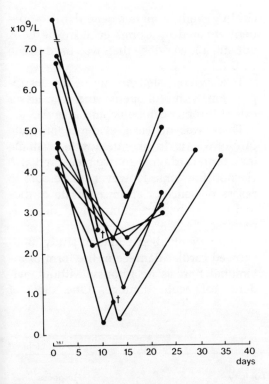

FIGURE 1. Effect of carminomycin on white blood cell counts.

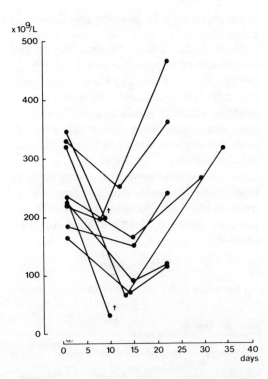

FIGURE 2. Effect of carminomycin on platelet counts.

anorexia and mild stomatitis were noted. Five patients complained of mild to moderate hair loss. Two patients complained of mild cutaneous radiation-recall reactions. No hepatic or renal toxicity was noted.

No ECG changes were seen prior to or following a dose of carminomycin, with two exceptions: Patient 5 died one month after the first dose of carminomycin due to congestive heart failure after pulmonary insufficiency with tumor infiltration and lymphangitis. At autopsy fibrosis of the endocardium and myocardium was found, most likely due to previous radiotherapy. Tumor was also found in the pericardium. Patient 7 died 12 days after the first dose of carminomycin due to a septic shock with a leukocyte count of 0.8×10^9/L. At autopsy similar fibrotic post radiation damage of the myocardium was found. Both patients had cardiac arrhythmias recorded prior to death, consisting of sinus arrhythmia in patient 5 and multiple premature atrial

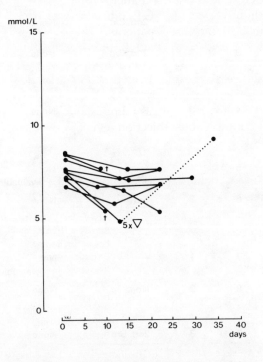

FIGURE 3. Effect of carminomycin on hemoglobin.

beats in patient 7. Results are shown in Table 2.

None of the other patients developed symptoms of congestive heart failure. In the patients 1, 2, 3, 4, 6, 8 and 9 we could evaluate left ventricular performance by ejection fraction studies, comparing the base line study with the result prior to each subsequent anthracycline treatment. Results are shown in Table 3.

No therapeutic responses were seen in these nine patients. Six patients subsequently received chemotherapy with doxorubicin. Three had stabilization of their disease.

Discussion

Our nine patients received carminomy-cin in a slightly higher dose than the patients treated by Comis et al in the USA but still a lower dose than was used in the USSR.

Toxicity consisted mainly of myelosuppression with leukopenia and to a lesser extent thrombocytopenia and anemia.

There was no clear evidence of acute cardiotoxicity. In an attempt to evaluate long term cardiotoxicity we measured also ejection fractions. However, to be able to assess presence or absence of late cardiotoxicity a higher cumulative dose is required.

Two patients died while on study. Both showed cardiac damage in the form of interstitial fibrosis at autopsy without evidence of acute damage. One died of

Table 2. Therapy

		Carminomycin			Doxorubicin
Patient	Nr of Courses	Dose Adjustments	Response	Toxicity	Response
1	2	2nd	None	Leukopenia Anorexia Headache	None
2	3	2nd, 3rd	None	Leukopenia Mild stomatitis	None
3	3	2nd, 3rd	None	Severe leukopenia, thrombocytopenia Mild stomatitis Moderate alopecia Mild radiation skin recall	—
4	3	3rd	None	Leukopenia, thrombocytopenia Moderate alopecia Mild radiation skin recall Slight headache	Stable
5	1	—	Not evaluable	Leukopenia	—
6	3	3rd	None	Leukopenia, thrombocytopenia Dry mouth Mild alopecia Mild somnolence	Stable
7	1	—	Not evaluable	Leukopenia, thrombocytopenia Stomatitis	—
8	2	None	None	Leukopenia Dry mouth Mild alopecia	None
9	3	2nd, 3rd	None	Leukopenia Mild alopecia Dizziness	Stable

Table 3. Ejection Fractions Prior to Each Course of Anthracycline

Patient	Baseline	CMM[a] II	CMM III	ADM I
1	0.72	0.68	–	0.73
2	0.61	0.48	0.46	0.52
3	0.75	0.71	0.54	
4	0.57	0.80	0.59	0.64
6	0.61	0.57	0.60	
8	0.56	0.51	–	0.47
9	0.55	0.73	0.51	0.57

[a]CMM: Carminomycin; ADM: Doxorubicin.

congestive heart failure accompanied by lymphangitis carcinomatosis, the other suffered septic shock.

Since no therapeutic response was seen in our patients they discontinued carminomycin therapy early and so evaluation of cardiac toxicity is of limited value.

Carminomycin in this regimen revealed in our experience only moderate acute toxicity and no therapeutic activity.

Further studies are recently concluded in the EORTC Soft Tissue and Bone Sarcoma Group and in advanced breast cancer in the EORTC Early Clinical Trials Group. These have confirmed the lack of activity of carminomycin. Evaluation of cardiotoxicity at high cumulative dosages awaits further study perhaps with a more optimal dosage schedule. The question of comparative cardiotoxicity is irrelevant if the drug is stopped early due to lack of tumor response.

ACKNOWLEDGMENTS

Thanks are due to the Queen Wilhelmina Funds (Project NKI 81/3) and the EORTC Pharmacokinetic and Metabolism, ECTG and Soft Tissue Sarcoma Groups.

REFERENCES

1. Gause, GF, Braznikova, MG, Shorin VA: *Cancer Chemother Rep 58: 255–256, 1974.*
2. Zbinden G, Branale E: *Cancer Chemother Rep 59: 707–715, 1975.*
3. Merski JA, Daskal Y, Crooke ST, Busch H: *Cancer Res 39: 1239–1244, 1979.*
4. Baker LH, Kessel DH, Comis RL, Reich SD, DeFuria MD, Crooke ST: *Cancer Treat Rep 63: 899–902, 1979.*
5. Comis RL, Ginsberg SJ, Reich SD, Baker LH, Crooke ST: New Drugs in Cancer Chemotherapy, Carter SK (Ed). Springer Verlag, Berlin/Heidelberg/New York, 1981 p. 16–20.
6. EORTC Soft Tissue and Bone Sarcoma Group: Proceedings of Third NCI-EORTC Symposium on New Drugs in Cancer Therapy, Brussels 1981.
7. EORTC Early Clinical Trials Group: Proceedings of Third NCI-EORTC Symposium on New Drugs in Cancer Therapy, Brussels 1981.
8. WHO Handbook for Reporting of Cancer Treatment: *Neoplasma 27: 607–619, 1980.*
9. Lankelma J, Penders PGM, McVie JG, Leyva A, ten Bokkel Huinink WW, de Planque MM, Pinedo HM: *Europ. J. Cancer and Clin Oncol.* In press.

CHAPTER 28

Diethoxyacetoxy Daunorubicin (Detorubicin)

M. Weil[a], Cl. Jacquillat[a], M. F. Auclerc[a], J. Maral[a], C. Bonnat[b], B. Diquet[b], and J. Khayat[b]

Experimental Data

The preparation and experimental antitumor activity of this new semi-synthetic compound was described by Maral et al. in 1978.[1,2]

Table 1 summarizes the differences in experimental activities between detorubicin and doxorubicin. These data are very encouraging and show that, although it may be considered as a prodrug of doxorubicin, detorubicin has different properties.

Clinical Activity

MATERIAL AND METHODS

We shall report here the results of phase I and II studies that we undertook between 1979 and 1980 in the Department of Hematology of the Hospital St-Louis, of which Professor Jean Bernard was the director.

Table 2 shows the diagnoses of the 139 patients. All were advanced cases: relapses of acute leukemia or metastatic

Table 1. Comparison of Experimental Activity of Detorubicin and Doxorubicin

Activity	Detorubicin Compared to Doxorubicin
Toxic	Less toxic
Cardiotoxic	Same range
Immunosuppressive	Less suppressive (Jernes' technique)
Mutagenic	Less (Ames test)
Experimental antitumor activity	For equitoxic doses chemotherapeutic index: equal or better (detorubicin 17.5-18.5; doxorubicin 14.1-15.0)
Experimental pharmacokinetic studies (mice)	Differences at cellular, plasma, and tissue levels

Table 2. Distribution of Diagnoses in 139 Patients Treated with Detorubicin

ALL	26
A.M.L.	9
Acute promyelocytic leukemia (M3)	3
Acute monoblastic leukemia (M5)	4
Acute phase of chronic myelogenous leukemia	5
Subtotal	47
Non-Hodgkin's lymphoma	25
Soft tissue sarcoma	4
Hodgkin's disease	4
Epithelioma	23
Malignant melanoma	1
Mesothelioma	1
Osteosarcoma	3
Ewing's sarcoma	1
Parker and Johnson	2
Mycosis fungoides	8
Subtotal	92
Total	139

[a]Service d'Oncologie Médicale, Hôpital de la Salpétrière, Service du Professeur Claude Jacquillat, Paris Cedex 13, France
[b]Département de Pharmacocinétique Clinique, Service des Professeurs Pierre Simon et Alain Thuillier, Paris Cedex 13, France

Table 3.   Toxicity of Detorubicin According to Various Schedules

Schedule	Gastrointestinal Toxicity				Hematologic Toxicity				Cardiotoxicity			
	1	2	3	4	1	2	3	4	1	2	3	4
2 mg/kg for 5 days		11	17	1			31	2				
2 mg/kg for 2 days (25 patients)	4	1				8	17					1
2 mg/kg every 3 weeks (49 patients)						35						1[a]
5 mg/kg								1				
1 mg/kg					7	1						

[a]After 30 mg/kg.

cancers, which were refractory to standard drug therapies. The drug was administered I.V. Schedules and doses varied according to diagnosis as follows:

1. In acute leukemias, courses of 5 sequential days: (2 mg/kg/day) mean total doses 12 mg/kg
2. In non-Hodgkin's lymphomas, 2 sequential days every 3 weeks (2 mg/kg/day)
3. In solid tumors, 2 mg/kg or 120 mg/m² every 2 or 3 weeks.

TOXICITY

The toxicity varied according to the posology, as shown in Table 3. Gastrointestinal toxicity of daily doses was exceedingly severe with ulceration, bowel pains, and diarrhea. Hematologic toxicity was severe with five daily doses or with two daily doses. One dose of 5 mg/kg induced irreversible aplasia, but intermittent doses of 120 mg/m² were well tolerated.

Two patients had cardiac toxicity. One dose of 4 mg/kg was followed by atrial fibrillation. One patient with melanoma skin metastases whose partial remission (PR) was maintained by intermittent doses of detorubicin (cumulative dose of 30 mg/kg within 6 months) died from cardiac failure.

RESULTS

Results in acute lymphocytic leukemia (ALL) are shown in Table 4. In one patient with Burkitt-type leukemia who was refractory to cyclophosphamide, vincristine,

Table 4.   Results of Detorubicin in ALL

	First Attack	First Relapse	Second Relapse	Total
CR	1	10	3	14
PR		2		2
Failure	2	2	4	8
Induction death		2	1	3
Total	3	16	8	27

prednisone, and daunorubicin, a short remission was achieved.

Table 5 shows results achieved in acute myelocytic leukemia (AML). In some cases of acute monoblastic leukemia (5) with skin involvement, detorubicin was combined with rubidazone, which induced a high rate of hematological remission but which did not prevent skin relapses.

In non-Hodgkin's lymphoma, we considered the complete disappearance of

Table 5.   Results of Detorubicin in Acute Myelocytic Leukemia

	AML (M1, M2, M4, M6)	Acute Promyelocytic Leukemia (M3)	Acute Monoblastic Leukemia (M5)	Total
CR	1	2	2	5
PR		1		1
Failure	6		1	7
Induction death	1		1	2
Total	8	3	4	15

clinical, hematologic, and radiologic disorders as a remission. However, since there was no surgical restaging, complete remission (CR) was not documented. As shown in Table 6, the rate of remission was 68%. Expecially impressive was the disappearance of bulky skin nodules, and the regression of mediastinal lymph nodes with pleural effusion and of the VII and XII cranial nerve palsy.

Table 6. Detorubicin in Non-Hodgkin's Lymphoma

	First Attack	Relapse or Failure of MOPP	Total
CR PR	4	13	17 (68%)
Failures	—	8	8
Total	4	21	25

Table 7 shows the results achieved by detorubicin in soft tissue sarcomas: Detorubicin like doxorubicin is an active drug in this case. In the one patient with melanoma already mentioned, regression of more than 50% was observed, but the patient died from cardiac failure after 6 months of treatment. In the other 15 patients, there was no result. In 7 of 8 patients with mycosis fungoids treated by 1 mg/kg of detorubicin once a week, regression of more than 50% was observed.

Table 7. Detorubicin in Soft Tissue Sarcomas

	CR	50% Regression	Failures
Rhabdomyosarcoma	1	1	
Liposarcoma		1	
Peritoneal mesothelioma		1	
Hemangiosarcoma			1

Table 8 shows the results observed in solid tumors refractory to standard drugs. They confirm the activity of detorubicin in solid tumors.

Pharmacokinetics

Plasma levels of detorubicin and doxorubicin after I.V. injection of 120 mg/m² of

Table 8. Results of Detorubicin in Solid Tumors

≥50% (3 patients)	Metastatic lymph node (thyroid)
	Metastatic skin nodules (kidney)
	Metastatic bone, local (kidney)
<50% (8 patients)	Lung metastasis (thyroid)
	Ovary (Stage IV)
	Lung epidermoid carcinoma
	Breast
	Hepatoma (alpha-fetoprotein)
Failures (9 patients)	Testis teratoma
	Tongue
	Ovary
	Skin metastasis (lung)
	Hepatoma

detorubicin are the results of either transformation of detorubicin to doxorubicin related to *in vivo* hydrolysis, or degradation of detorubicin into doxorubicin related to the method used: 1) solubilization in distilled water before injection at pH 5,8, the half-life values of hydrolysis being 88 minutes,[3] 2) light exposure and room temperature before and during injection, and 3) blood sample extraction.

To investigate pharmacokinetic parameters of detorubicin in plasma, we measured, on the one hand, detorubicin and doxorubicin in blood samples (collected on citrate buffer, 0.2 M immediatly centrifuged and frozen), and, on the other, doxorubicin related to analytical assay, in order to correct the measured plasma half-life. It is very important to point out that, if no care is taken, detorubicin is no longer detectable after 10 minutes.

Detorubicin and doxorubicin are detected in plasma by high pressure liquid chromotography (HPLC), on a RP 18 column with acetonitrile-formate buffer-MgCl$_2$ solvent (635-335-30) at a flow rate of 3.5 mg/mn, injection valve with a 100 μl loop, and fluorimetric detection (E = 470 nm, F = 551 nm). Extraction procedure was performed as described by Robert,[4] using C$_{18}$ Sep-pak. Blood samples were collected a very short time after the injection (1, 2, 3, 5, 10, 15, 30, 60 minutes). Patients had not received anthracycline treatment before the assay.

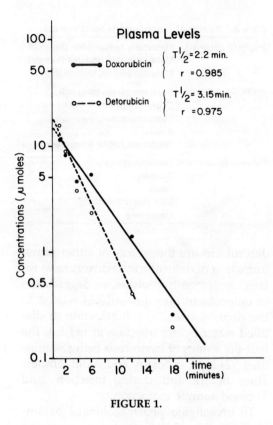

FIGURE 1.

Conclusion

These data confirm that the detorubicin spectrum of activity is very close to that of doxorubicin. Since there is a rapid transformation of detorubicin to doxorubicin in plasma,[3] one may ask if detorubicin is really different from doxorubicin. We have already mentioned that, in mice, there are differences in cellular accumulation between these two drugs.

Preliminary pharmacokinetic study in human beings suggests differences between the two drugs.

Clinical results indicate preferential accumulation of the drug in the skin and in the gastrointestinal tract. Further studies are required.

ACKNOWLEDGMENTS

This work was supported by INSERM Contract, Commission 8 (Prof. Laudat); Franco-American Committee for Research on Cancer (INSERM); USPHS Research Grant, CA 13 239-05, National Cancer Institute; and Unit 232, INSERM.

Results

Figure 1 shows plasma levels of detorubicin and doxorubicin in one patient. Plasma half-lives corresponding to the first elimination phase were 2.2 minutes for detorubicin and 3.15 minutes for doxorubicin.

The apparent volume of distribution of doxorubicin (as detorubicin degradation result) seems to be different from the volume of distribution following doxorubicin I.V. injection.[5] This leads to a similar hypothesis published by Deprez-de Campeneere et al.[3] studying tissue distribution of detorubicin related to doxorubin.

These observations are preliminary results and need to be confirmed on a larger group of patients.

REFERENCES

1. Maral R, Ducep J, Fargues BD, Ponsinet G, Reisdorf D: Preparation and experimental antitumor activity of a new semi-synthetic compound: 14-Diethoxyacetoxy daunorubicin (RP 33 921). CR Acad Sci [D] (Paris), 286(5): 443-446, 1978.
2. Maral R: Comparative study of detorubicin and doxorubicin (adriamycin). Am Assoc Cancer Res 20: 116, 1979.
3. Deprez-de Campeneere D, Baurain R, Trouet A: Pharmacokinetic, toxicology and chemotherapeutic properties of detorubicin in mice: A comparative study with daunorubicin and adriamycin. Cancer Treat Rep 64(5):861-867, 1979.
4. Robert J: Extraction of anthracyclines from biological fluids for HPLC evaluation. J Chromatogr 3(10): 1561-1572, 1980.
5. Benjamin RS, Riggs CE Jr, Bachur NR: Plasma pharmacokinetics of adriamycin and its metabolites in humans. Cancer Res 37: 1416, 1977.

Part VII

Clinical Studies
Candidates for Phase I Trials

N-L-Leucyl Derivatives of Daunorubicin and Doxorubicin as New Prodrugs of Anthracyclines

A. Trouet, D. Deprez-De Campeneere, R. Baurain, and M. Masquelier

We have recently synthesized and studied N-amino acid and dipeptide derivatives of daunorubicin (DNR) as potential prodrugs of this antitumor agent.[1] It was assumed that such prodrugs could have different pharmacokinetic properties and could regenerate DNR inside tumor cells or in their vicinity after enzymatic hydrolysis. Among these derivatives, L-leucyl-DNR (LEU-DNR) was found to be the most interesting. We have therefore studied more extensively the toxicologic, pharmacokinetic, and therapeutic properties of the the N-L-leucyl derivatives of DNR and doxorubicin (DOX).

As compared to their parent anthracyclines, LEU-DNR and LEU-DOX are characterized by a fourfold decreased overall toxicity as determined in terms of mortality in mice after I.V. administration (Table 1). Both derivatives after single I.V. injection are about three times less toxic for the bone marrow pluripotent (colony-forming units-spleen [CFU-S] assay) and myeloid committed (colony-forming units-culture [CFU-C] assay) stem cells. The decreased toxicity observed with LEU-DNR and LEU-DOX after I.V. injection goes in parallel with a lower accumulation of these drugs in several tissues, mainly in the cardiac muscle.

Table 1. Compared Toxicity of Daunorubicin, Doxorubicin, and Their L-Leucyl Derivatives: LD50 Study

Drug	LD_{50}[a] (mg/kg/day)
DNR	16.8 ± 1.2
LEU-DNR	67.0 ± 1.8
DOX	14.4 ± 2.3
LEU-DOX	46.7 ± 1.8

[a]LD_{50} is a dose that induces 50% lethality in mice after 30 days of observation. Drugs were administered I.V. on two consecutive days. Mean $\pm$ S.D. of two (L-leucyl derivatives) or three separate assays are given.

A chronic study performed in the rabbit has also outlined the lower hematotoxicity of LEU-DNR and LEU-DOX. The histopathologic evaluation of the chronic cardiotoxicity[3] has shown that LEU-DNR and LEU-DOX given, respectively, at 3.5 and 3 times the dosage of DNR or DOX were markedly less cardiotoxic than the parent compounds after 11 or 16 weeks of I.V. treatment. The most striking difference was noted with LEU-DNR, which showed significantly less myocardial disease than did DNR in spite of the higher doses given.

We have obtained, moreover, pharmacokinetic data[3] that correlate well with the results of the chronic cardiotoxicity. After a single I.V. injection at equimolar doses, the total drug level reached in rabbit heart as a function of time was much lower after administration of LEU-DNR and LEU-

International Institute of Cellular and Molecular Pathology and Université Catholique de Louvain, Brussels, Belgium

DOX as compared to DNR or DOX. The difference observed in chronic cardiotoxicity between LEU-DNR and LEU-DOX, the latter drug being more toxic for the heart than the former, may be attributed to a difference in enzymatic hydrolysis of the drugs into their parent anthracyclines. This explanation is supported by two features. First, the amount of DOX found in rabbit heart after I.V. injection LEU-DOX is greater than the amount of DNR found after LEU-DNR injection. Second, as assayed *in vitro* on heart homogenates, LEU-DOX is much more hydrolyzed than LEU-DNR in its parent compound; the enzyme responsible for this hydrolysis in the heart having a greater affinity for LEU-DOX as substrate with an optimal activity at pH 7.

Finally, as illustrated in Table 2, both leucyl derivatives have been studied for their therapeutic effectiveness on murine L1210 leukemia. When both leukemic cells and drugs are given I.V. at equitoxic doses, the leucyl derivatives are less active than their parent drugs. In contrast, after I.V. administration at equitoxic doses, LEU-DNR and LEU-DOX exert a striking activity on the intraperitoneal and subcutaneous forms of L1210 leukemia, as indicated by the high percentage of mice surviving on day 30 and by the important reduction in tumor development in the case of subcutaneously implanted L1210 cells.

In an attempt to understand this peculiar therapeutic effect and the mode of activation of the leucyl derivatives, we have followed the drug accumulation and metabolism of LEU-DNR in diffusion chambers[2] implanted subcutaneously or intraperitoneally in mice. Using this experimental system, we have found that after single I.V. injection at equimolar doses, LEU-DNR accumulates at higher levels than DNR and undergoes a slow hydrolysis into DNR.

In conclusion, LEU-DNR and LEU-DOX, weakly active as such, possess over their parent anthracyclines the great advantage of a decreased toxicity in terms of mortality, hematopoietic toxicity, and cardiotoxicity, the last point being the most important one, especially for LEU-DNR. After I.V. administration, the leucyl derivatives seem to reach more easily the subcutaneous tissue and the peritoneal cavity,

Table 2. Chemotherapeutic Activity of N-L-Leucyl Derivatives of Daunorubicin and Doxorubicin on Murine L1210 Leukemia

L1210 Cells[a]	Route	Drug	Doses, mg/kg/day	Increase in Life-span (%)	No. of Survivors on Day 30/ Total No. of Mice	Average Tumor Diameter (mm)	
						Day 8	Day 12
10^4	I.P.	DNR	11	88	1/29	–	–
10^4	I.P.	DOX	6	120	2/10	–	–
10^4	I.P.	LEU-DNR	44	>247	13/19	–	–
10^4	I.P.	LEU-DOX	20	>233	5/9	–	–
10^4	I.V.	DNR	11	66	0/37	–	–
10^4	I.V.	DOX	7	76	4/25	–	–
10^4	I.V.	LEU-DNR	44	39	0/7	–	–
10^4	I.V.	LEU-DOX	24	40	0/8	–	–
10^5	S.C.	DNR	11	67	3/37	0.4	2.9
10^5	S.C.	DOX	7	234	19/27	0	0
10^5	S.C.	LEU-DNR	44	215	14/25	0	0.1
10^5	S.C.	LEU-DOX	24	>228	20/29	0	0.1

[a]L1210 cells were inoculated on day 0 into DBA/2 mice. Drugs were given I.V. on days 1 and 2 at equitoxic doses.

probably because of their greater lipophilicity than DNR or DOX. The enhanced chemotherapeutic activities observed with these derivatives on the subcutaneous and intraperitoneal forms of L1210 leukemia could therefore be explained by the higher drug concentration reached at the target sites and by a consecutive enzymatic hydrolysis into the parent drug. The L-leucyl derivatives of anthracyclines can thus be considered as promising new prodrugs.

REFERENCES

1. Baurain R, Masquelier M, Deprez-De Campeneere D, Trouet A: Amino acid and dipeptide derivatives of daunorubicin. 2. Cellular pharmacology and antitumor activity on L1210 leukemic cells *in vitro* and *in vivo. J Med Chem 23: 1171-1174, 1980.*
2. Huybrechts M, Symann M, Trouet A: The diffusion chamber technique as an *in vivo* assay in mice for the effectiveness of antitumor agents. *Scand J Haematol 23: 223-226, 1979.*
3. Jaenke RS, Deprez-De Campeneere D, Trouet A: Cardiotoxicity and comparative pharmacokinetics of six anthracyclines in the rabbit. *Cancer Res 40: 3530-3536, 1980.*

CHAPTER 30

Comparative Experimental Studies on 4'-O-Tetrahydropyranyl-Adriamycin and Adriamycin

H. Umezawa,[a] K. Yamada[b] and T. Oki[c]

The significant therapeutic advantages gained by the structural difference at C-4' position between daunomycin (DM) and baumycin Al has led us to prepare 4'-O-glycosidic derivatives of adriamycin (ADM) and DM.

In the screening of antitumor anthracycline glycosides with lower toxicity and superior antitumor activity than the ADM, new members of the DM group of antibiotics, the baumycins, have been isolated from the culture broth of *Streptomyces coeruleorubidus* ME130-A4.[1,2] In the preliminary test of the antitumor activity against L1210 leukemia, baumycin Al (Fig. 1) exhibited stronger activity and potency than ADM and DM. Because of its low yield for production and unreliability in activity, consequently we decided to synthesize the simple 4'-O-glycosidic derivatives and evaluate their antitumor activity against L1210 leukemia. As shown in Table 1, among tetrahydropyranyl and tetrahydrofuranyl derivatives of ADM and DM, 4'-O-tetrahydropyranyladriamycin (b) (THP-ADM) was most active and superior to ADM.[3] Comparative biologic, toxicologic and pharmacologic studies on THP-ADM and ADM are reviewed in this chapter.

[a]Institute of Microbial Chemistry, Tokyo
[b]First Department Internal Medicine, Nagoya University School of Medicine, Nagoya
[c]Central Research Laboratories, Sanraku Ocean Co., Fujisawa, Japan

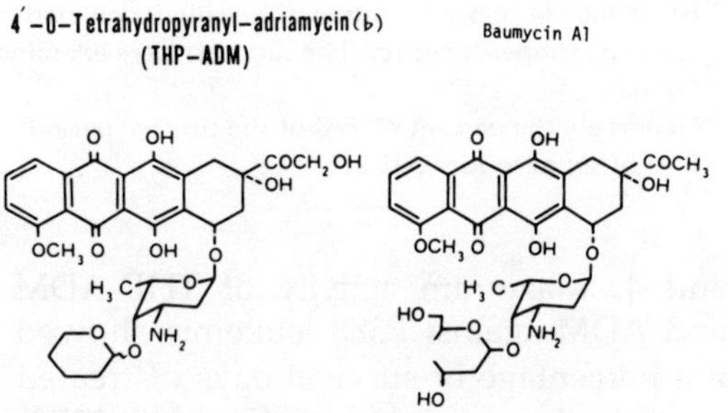

FIGURE 1. Chemical structure.

Antitumor Activity

Inhibitory effects of THP-ADM and related anthracyclines on the growth and macromolecular biosynthesis of cultured L1210 leukemia cells were expressed as the IC_{50} (50% inhibition concentration, μg/ml) values, which determined using probit analysis, as shown in Table 2, When the IC_{50} (50% inhibition concentration, μg/ml values, IC_{50} values of THP-ADM, ADM, and DM were compared, THP-ADM was twice as cytotoxic as ADM and DM and inhibited both RNA and DNA synthesis at about a 10-fold lower concentration than that of DM. THP-ADM was mutagenic in the Ames system. In addition, THP-ADM was more active against a variety of murine tumors than ADM.

The antitumor activity of THP-ADM was superior to that of ADM against P388 and L1210 leukemias, as shown in Tables 3

Table 1. Antitumor Activity of Tetrahydropyranyl and Tetrahydrofuranyl Derivatives of Daunomycin and Adriamycin Against L1210 Leukemia[a]

	Dose (mg/kg/day)					
Compounds	5	2.5	1.25	0.63	0.31	0.16
DM	Toxic	138[b,c]	191	145	132	118
4'-O-Tetrahydropyranyl DM(a)	320[b]	474	122	115	96	90
4'-O-Tetrahydropyranyl DM(b)	320[b]	256	122	115	103	90
ADM	180[b]	458	278	373	198	131
14,4'-O-Ditetrahydropyranyl ADM(a)	154	115	109	96	103	96
14,4'-O-Ditetrahydropyranyl ADM(b)	161	109	103	103	96	115
14-O-Tetrahydropyranyl ADM	142	130	126	113	110	103
4'-O-Tetrahydropyranyl ADM(a)	–	173	180	187	120	127
4'-O-Tetrahydropyranyl ADM(b)	800[d]	473	427	342	171	129
4'-O-Tetrahydrofuranyl ADM(a)	212[b]	288	189	135	115	115
4'-O-Tetrahydrofuranyl ADM(b)	256[b]	230	154	141	128	122

[a]10^5 leukemia cells were intraperitoneally inoculated in CDF_1 mice. Compounds were daily administered from day 1–9 intraperitoneally. The survivals were examined up to 60 days.
[b]Toxic.
[c]Figures are the percent of T/C of the survival period.
[d]Five of six mice survived.

and 4. Maximum activity of THP-ADM and ADM against P388 leukemia showed the percentage of survival days of treated group to those of control (T/C) of 245–257% and 241–247%, respectively, at the daily dose of 1.25–2.5 mg/kg for 10 days. Two, 5, and 1 out of 12 mice treated with 5, 2.5, and 1.25 mg/kg/day of THP-ADM, respectively were tumor-free, whereas ADM showed no survivors on the 60-day observation. Superior antitumor effect of THP-ADM to ADM was observed in the intravenous and intraperitoneal administration of 12.5 mg/kg on day 1, and 6.25 mg/kg on

day 1 and 2 or day 1 and 3 against L1210 leukemia. Intravenous THP-ADM gave two and four survivors out of six mice, but there were no survivors with intravenous ADM.

The effects of THP-ADM against subcutaneously implanted B16 melanoma and colon 38 and intraperitoneally implanted colon 26 were examined by five times the intraperitoneal administration every other day starting from 1 day after implantation, and the results are summarized in Table 5. ADM did not show therapeutic responses against colon 38 and B16 melanoma, where-

Table 2. Inhibitory Effects of THP-Adriamycin and Related Anthracyclines on the Growth and Macromolecular Biosynthesis of Cultured L1210 Leukemia Cells

	IC_{50} (µg/ml)			
Anthracycline	Cell Growth	DNA Synthesis	RNA Synthesis	DNA/ RNA
THP-Adriamycin	0.01	0.12	0.06	2.0
Adriamycin	0.02	1.40	0.55	2.5
Daunomycin	0.02	0.42	0.16	2.6
Aclacinomycin A	0.01	0.30	0.038	7.9

Table 3. Antitumor Effect of THP-ADM and ADM Against P388 Leukemia[a]

	THP-ADM		ADM	
Dose[b] (mg/kg/day)	T/C (%)	60-Day Survivors	T/C (%)	60-Day Survivors
5.0	149	2/12	73	0/12
2.5	257	5/12	247	0/12
1.25	245	1/12	241	0/12
0.625	183	0/12	201	0/12

[a]Each group of 12 CDF_1 mice were given intraperitoneal implants of 10^6 cells on day 0.
[b]Drug was given I.P. every day for 10 days starting from day 1.

Table 4. Antitumor Effect of THP-ADM and ADM Against L1210 Leukemia[a]

Admini-stration Route	Schedule	THP-ADM		ADM	
		T/C (%)	60-Day Survivors	T/C (%)	60-Day Survivors
I.P.	Day 1	490	6/6	220	3/6
I.P.	Day 1 & 2	392	5/6	218	1/6
I.P.	Day 1 & 3	322	3/6	273	3/6
I.V.	Day 1	217	4/6	192	0/6
I.V.	Day 1 & 2	283	4/6	213	0/6
I.V.	Day 1 & 3	246	2/6	172	0/6

[a]Each group of six CDF$_1$ mice was given intraperitoneal implants of 10^5 cells.

Dose: 12.5 mg/kg on Day 1; 6.25 mg/kg on Days 1 & 2 or 1 & 3.

Table 5. Antitumor Effect of THP-ADM and ADM Against B16 Melanoma (S.C.), Colon 26(I.P.), and Colon 38(S.C.)

Drug[a]	Dose (mg/kg)	T/C (%)[b]		
		B16 Mela-noma	Colon 26	Colon 38
THP-ADM	5.0	139[c]	195[d] (2/10)[e]	142
	2.5	93	161[d] (2/10)	134
	1.25	104	149[d] (1/10)	117
ADM	5.0	56	68	36
	2.5	97	188[d] (8/10)	84
	1.25	92	205[d] (5/10)	94

[a]Drug was given intraperitoneally every 2 days for five days from day 1.
[b]B16 melanoma and colon adenocarcinoma 38 were implanted subcutaneously into the flank of BDF$_1$ mice. Colon adenocarcinoma 26 were implanted intraperitoneally into CDF$_1$ mice.
[c]$P < 0.05$ by Student's t-test.
[d]$P < 0.05$ by U test.
[e]Number in parenthesis: 90-day survivors/number of treated mice.

Table 6. Inhibition of Lewis Lung Carcinoma by THP-ADM and ADM[a]

Drug	Dose (mg/kg)	T/C (%)	Lung Metastasis[b]
Experiment 1 (every 2 days for 5 days from day 1)			
THP-ADM	7.5	82 (1/10)[c]	—
	5.0	158[d]	0.5 ± 0.3 (1.1)[d]
	2.5	116	9.4 ± 1.9 (20.1)[d]
	1.25	111	18.6 ± 3.5 (39.8)[d]
ADM	2.5	78	15.6 ± 4.2 (33.4)[d]
	1.25	127	37.5 ± 5.0 (80.3)
	0.63	105	40.0 ± 5.0 (91.4)
Experiment 2 (every 2 days for 5 days from day 7)			
THP-ADM	7.5	82	—
	5.0	138[d]	4.8 ± 1.5 (10.3)[d]
	2.5	123	14.6 ± 3.3 (31.3)[d]
	1.25	114	26.5 ± 6.6 (56.7)[d]
ADM	2.5	79	44.6 ± 7.0 (95.5)
	1.25	111	40.8 ± 9.7 (87.4)
	0.63	103	44.0 ± 5.0 (94.2)
Control		100	46.7 ± 4.4 (100)

[a]Each group of 20 BDF$_1$ mice was implanted subcutaneously with 5×10^5 cells of dissociated Lewis lung carcinoma on day 0.
[b]Lung metastases of 10 mice from each group were counted on day 21. The value in the parenthesis represents percent of the control tumor nodules.
[c]Number in parenthesis: 90-day survivors/number of treated mice.
[d]$P < 0.05$ by Student's t test.

as significant effects were obtained at 5 mg/kg of THP-ADM against B16 (T/C = 139%) and colon 38 (T/C = 142%). Both drugs showed good therapeutic effect on colon 26, and ADM was more effective with more than THP-ADM.

Against subcutaneous Lewis lung carcinoma, THP-ADM and ADM were given intraperitoneally five times every other day, starting from day 1 (experiment 1: early stage of tumor development) or day 7 (experiment 2: advanced stage of tumor development) after implantation, and a T/C and lung metastasis were examined on day 90 and 21, respectively. In experiment 1, a maximum T/C of 158% was obtained with 5 mg/kg THP-ADM, but ADM gave only 127% T/C at 1.25 mg/kg, and the dose of 2.5 mg/kg was toxic. This shows that THP-ADM is more than three times less toxic than ADM. Against the advanced stage of Lewis lung carcinoma, 5 mg/kg THP-ADM showed a maximum T/C of 138%, but no significant therapeutic response was observed with ADM (Table 6).

Furthermore, THP-ADM inhibited remarkably the lung metastasis of Lewis lung carcinoma. In the control group, an average of 46.7 of macroscopically countable tumor nodules was observed in the lung on day 21. At the most effective dose of 5 mg/kg of THP-ADM, the number of tumor nodules in the lung was reduced to less than 10% that of the controls in the early and advanced stages of tumor development. ADM, however, had only a marginal effect on the lung metastasis. As described later, it seems that very high distribution of THP-ADM in the lung relates to the marked inhibition on lung metastasis of Lewis lung carcinoma.

Toxicity[6] and Cardiotoxicity[4]

LD_{50} values of THP-ADM were calculated by mortality on a 14-day observation based on the Litchfield and Wilcoxon method. The LD_{50} values of THP-ADM in dd mice after a single I.V., I.P., or S.C. dose ranged from 17 to 26 mg/kg, as shown in Table 7, and about two to three times higher than the values reported on ADM. Dogs administered 2.5 mg/kg ADM intravenously showed slight and transient scratching of the skin and edema of the facial skin immediately after the injection. However, these abnormalities were not observed in the THP-ADM-treated dogs with 2.5 mg/kg intravenously. Other toxic symptoms in dogs commonly caused by the two drugs were loss of weight, vomiting, diarrhea, bloody excrement, hemorrhage in the gastrointestinal tract and slight changes in electrocardiogram (ECG) just after the injection. A decrease in the white blood cell count was a little heavier in the THP-ADM-treated dogs than in the ADM-treated animals.

The electron microscopic (EM) study by Mathé et al.[4] of the myocardium of the THP-ADM-treated golden hamsters at the end of the first and second weeks of treatment with the dose of 4 mg/kg, three times a week, showed very rare and mild lesions; some myocytes had swelling of the mitochondria, clearing of their matrices, and lysis of the crests, but most mitochondria, myofilaments, and intercalated disks were well preserved. Two months after THP-ADM treatment had been stopped, there was a recovery in the myocardial EM changes. On the other hand, the myocardium of animals treated with ADM showed very severe EM alterations. Mathé concluded that THP-ADM is the least cardiotoxic and far less toxic on the skin than any anthracyclines being used at present. In our experiments, acute ECG changes with THP-ADM and ADM was comparatively examined in golden hamsters after a single intravenous administration, monitoring by the standard lead II. Administration of 3 mg/kg of ADM produced slight ECG changes in 4 of 5 hamsters and 6 mg/kg cauused marked abnormalities on ECG in all animals, whereas 6 mg/kg of THP-ADM caused only slight arrhythmia comparable to that of 1.5 mg/kg of ADM. Accordingly, the acute cardiotoxicity of THP-ADM was found to be significantly lower than that of ADM.

Pharmacology[6]

Metabolism of THP-ADM was examined with liver homogenates of rats and dogs using high performance liquid chromatography. In the reaction mixture containing liver homogenate in phosphate-buffered saline (pH 7), 2 μg/ml of THP-ADM, 0.5 mM of NADPH, and 0.5 mM NADH at 37°C in nitrogen gas, THP-ADM was converted to 4'-O-tetrahydropyranyladriamycinol (THP-ADM-OH) by aldo-keto reductase at the C-13 position of adriamycinone with small extent, and then extensively degraded to the aglycone-type metabolites; 7-deoxyadriamycinone and 7-deoxy-13-dihydroadriamycinone by NADPH-cytochrome P-450 reductase in the liver homog-

Table 7.   Acute Toxicity of THP-ADM in Mice

Administration Route	LD_{50} (mg/kg) Male
I.V.	24.00 (22.96–25.04)[a]
I.P.	17.89 (16.85–18.92)
S.C.	26.61 (25.57–27.65)

[a]Confidence limit of 95%.

enate through the reductive glycosidic cleavage at the C-7 position of glycosides. The resulting aglycone metabolites seem to be resolubilized further by conjugation with glucuronic acid and with sulfate to be excreted in the urine. Adriamycin was not detected under this reaction condition. The cleavage of THP residue was slightly caused by mouse and dog liver homogenates in acetate buffer at pH 5.0 without NADH and NADPH. Hydrolysis at C-4' position to release ADM seems very unlikely *in vivo*, because ADM was detected in only small amount in the blood, urine, and various tissues. Therefore, proposed metabolic pathway of THP-ADM is deduced, as shown in Figure 2.

The plasma level and clearance of THP-ADM and ADM in dogs were examined by an intravenous injection of 1.5 mg/kg. As shown in Figure 3, plasma levels of both drugs decreased rapidly and remained nearly constant at a low level for a long period of time. Pharmacokinetic parameters of THP-ADM and ADM in dogs were calculated, based on a three compartment model by successive linear regression analysis. The three successive half-lives were 0.07 hour, 0.5 hour, and 8.5 hours for THP-ADM and 0.04 hour, 0.25 hour, and 5.4 hours for ADM. The relative

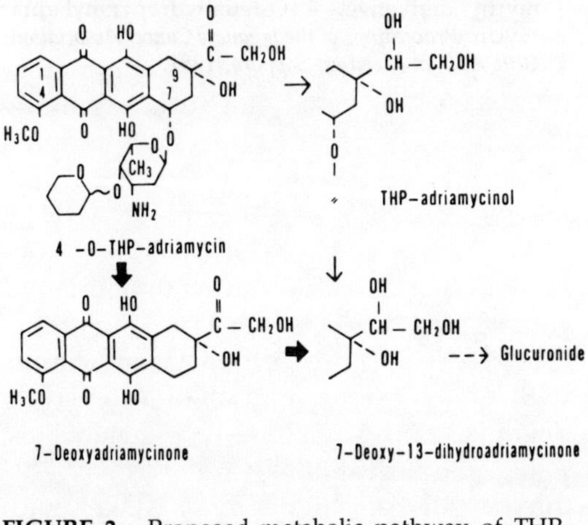

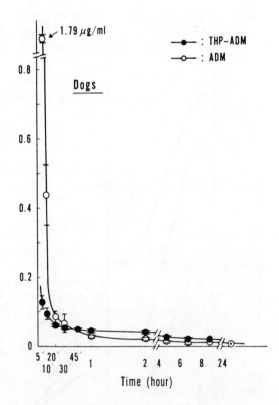

FIGURE 3. Plasma levels of ADM and THP-ADM in dogs. Dose: 1.5 mg/kg, $n = 4$, intravenously.

volume of distribution (Vd) of the three compartments were in contrast highly different from THP-ADM (42 liter/kg) to ADM (6.6 liter/kg).

Cumulative excretion of the parent drug and its metabolites, which were extracted with chloroform-methanol (2:1) mixture at pH 9, into the urine was about 3% within 70 hours in the ADM-treated dogs, but only about 1% of the injected THP-ADM was recovered in the urine. More polar metabolites, including the conjugated metabolites, should be further analyzed.

Tissue distributions of THP-ADM and ADM in dogs 2 and 8 hours after the administration of a dose of 1.5 mg/kg intravenously are shown in Figure 4. Initially, the concentration of THP-ADM was greater than that of ADM in the spleen, lung, and thymus, and the levels in most

FIGURE 2. Proposed metabolic pathway of THP-ADM in mammals.

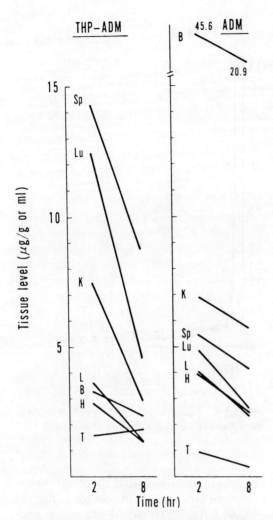

FIGURE 4. Tissue levels of ADM and THP-ADM administered intravenously in dogs (1.5 mg/kg). B: bile; K: kidney; Sp: spleen; Lu: lung; L: liver; H: heart; T: thymus.

organs decreased rapidly after 2 hours. In contrast, ADM was detected in the bile at an extremely high concentration, more in the heart and retained with smaller decay than THP-ADM. Thus, tissue distribution patterns and pharmacokinetics of THP-ADM differ considerably from those of ADM.

Clinical trial of THP-ADM is going to start soon in Japan after the chronic toxicity test in dogs is completed.

REFERENCES

1. Komiyama T, Matsuzawa Y, Oki T, Inui T, Taka-hashi Y, Naganawa H, Takeuchi T, Umezawa H: Baumycins, new antitumor antibiotics related to daunomycin. *J Antibiot (Tokyo)* 30: 619–621, 1977.
2. Takahashi Y, Naganawa H, Takeuchi T, Umezawa H, Komiyama T, Oki T, Inui T: The structure of baumycins A1, A2, B1, B2, C1 and C2. *J Antibiot (Tokyo)* 30: 622–624, 1977.
3. Umezawa H, Takahashi Y, Kinoshita M, Naganawa H, Masuda T, Ishizuka M, Tatsuta K, Takeuchi T: Tetrahydropyranyl derivatives of daunomycin and adriamycin. *J Antibiot (Tokyo)* 32: 1082–1084, 1979.
4. Dantchev D, Paintrand M, Hayat M, Bourut C, Mathé G: Low heart and skin toxicity of a tetra-hydropyranyl derivative of adriamycin (THP-ADM) as observed by electron and light micros-copy. *J Antibiot (Tokyo)* 32: 1085–1086, 1979.
5. Tsuruo T: Antitumor activity of tetrahydropyranyl derivative of adriamycin. *Cancer Chemother 8:* 179–181, 1980.
6. Iguchi H, Matsushita Y, Kiyoshima T, Tone H, Oki T, Ishikura T, Takeuchi T, Umezawa H: Antitumor activity and pharmacodynamics of a new adria-mycin derivative, 4'-O-tetrahydropyranyladria-mycin. *Proceedings of the Japanese Cancer Association, 40th Annual Meeting, Sapporo, 1981.*

CHAPTER 31

Rubicyclamine: Experimental Study

R. Maral, L. Julou, C. G. Caillard, S. Mondot, J. Pasquet, and P. Ganter

Among the daunorubicin (DNR) analogues (DNR chlorhydrate, MW: 563.9), the substitution of the daunosamine moiety by a six-membered ring, with an amine function displaying the same geometry as in the DNR molecule, was made with the hope of obtaining less cardiotoxic compounds.[1] Four isomers (cis A and B, trans A and B) correspond to the aminocyclohexane carboxylic esters of daunomycinone (Fig. 1).

The chlorhydrate salts of the isomers (MW: 560.0) are water soluble.

The choice of the more active isomer was made in various experimental tumor systems, namely, in L1210 leukemia; the more active compound was cis A ; this derivative was called rubicyclamin (RCA).

The experimental activity of RCA was compared with that of DNR.

Cytotoxicity in Cell Culture

KB cells were cultured in RPMI 1640 medium (supplemented with 10% calf serum) containing increasing concentrations of drugs; the cells were counted 3 days later and the inhibiting concentration (IC_{50}) was determined. The IC_{50} ($\mu g/ml$) for RCA was 0.930 and for DNR, 0.450.

In this system, the toxicity ratio between the two drugs was only 2, whereas in other systems, as will be seen later, the ratio was usually much higher.

Rhône-Poulenc Industries, Centre de Recherches Nicolas Grillet, Vitry-sur-Seine, France

DIFFUSION IN AGAR CHABBERT'S TECHNIQUE[2]

The two curves correlating the diameters of the cell inhibition and the drug concentrations were nonparallel straight lines. The concentrations giving an inhibition area of 20 mm diameter were 5.0 mg/ml for RCA and 0.35 mg/ml for DNR. The activity ratio was 14.

ACTIVITY ON DNA SYNTHESIS

The effect of the drug on the incorporation of tritiated thymidine in KB cells was studied. The precursor was added 1 hour before the cell harvest for counting. The ratios of treated cells to controls were plotted at different times. RCA inhibits the thymidine incorporation, but the kinetics of the inhibition is much slower.

ACTIVITY ON VIRUS MULTIPLICATION

At about 10 times the concentration of DNR, RCA inhibited (50%) the replication in cell culture of two DNA viruses: vaccinia (RCA: 3.6 $\mu g/ml$; DNR: 0.3 $\mu g/ml$) and myxomatosis virus (RCA: 7.2 $\mu g/ml$; DNR: 0.6 $\mu g/ml$).

Conversely, on an RNA virus (VSV), both compounds were inactive.

Toxicity in Mice

OF$_1$ or CD-1 adult mice, 10 animals per dose, were treated. The mice were observed for 21 days following the treatment.

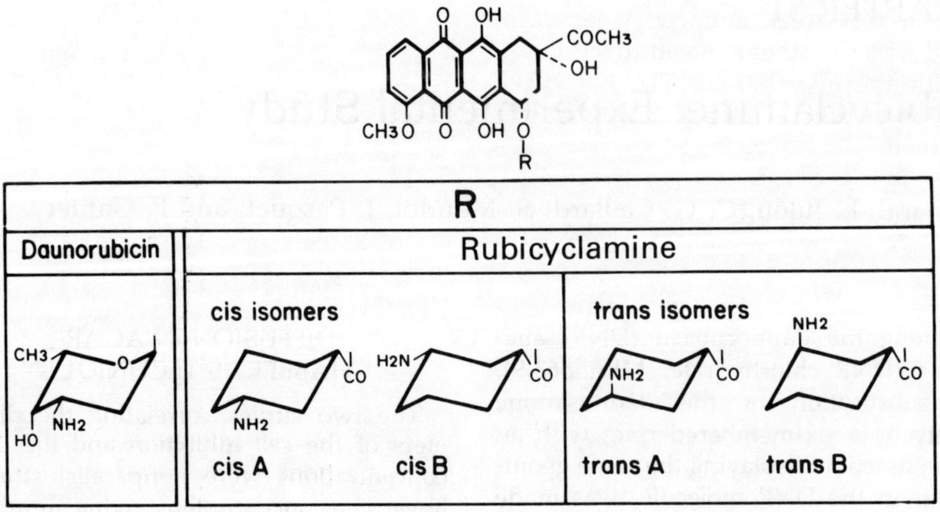

FIGURE 1.

ACUTE TOXICITY

RCA is about 5–10 times less toxic than DNR, by the I.P. or I.V. routes.

SUBACUTE TOXICITY

The mice were treated during 5 consecutive days. The results show that the comparative toxicity RCA/DNR depends on the route of treatment: by S.C. route, RCA (LD_{50}: 55 mg/kg S.C.) is about four to eight times less toxic ; by I.P. route, RCA (LD_{50}: 21 mg/kg I.P.) is about 10 times less toxic, and by I.V. route, RCA (LD_{50}: 23 mg/kg I.V.) is about three to four times less toxic.

Toxicity in Rabbits and Dogs

Fauve de Bourgogne rabbits, 4 months old, and beagle dogs, 10 to 12 months old, were used in this 1-month treatment study. The animals were treated for 5 days each week at the daily dose of 1, 2, 4, 8, and 16 mg/kg I.V. in the rabbit and, 0.5, 1, 2, 4, and 8 mg/kg I.V. in the dog.

Although the similar toxicologic study of DNR was performed long before that of RCA, we may conclude that RCA is about eight times less toxic than DNR.

Cardiac Toxicity

G. ZBINDEN'S TECHNIQUE[3]

The drugs were administered to rats by the I.P. route at the daily doses of 4 mg/kg for DNR and 10 and 20 mg/kg for RCA. The cardiotoxic action was considered positive when the QRS interval was lengthened by at least 15%. The cumulative cardiotoxic dose 50 (CCD_{50}) is the total dose that induced a cardiotoxic effect in 50% of the animals. The CCD_{50} intraperitoneally for RCA was 60-80 mg/kg and for DNR, 16 mg/kg. RCA is four to five times less cardiotoxic than DNR in this system.

D. DANTCHEV'S TECHNIQUE

Heart electron microscopy in the hamster showed that RCA is a weak cardiotoxic derivative. No important alopecia was observed in the animals.

Mutagenic Activity

Using the Ames technique[5], with the TA-98 strain of Salmonella typhimurium (his-) (frameshift mutation), RCA (0.1 n. mole to 5000 n. moles per plate) was found to be a very weak mutagen when compared with the other main anthracyclines.

With the other strains (TA-100, 1535, 1537, and 1538), no mutagenic activity was observed.

Immunopharmacology

RCA exerted no significant depressive activity on the carbon clearance test in mice.

With Jerne's technique (hemolytic plaques in gel produced by spleen cells), at equitoxic doses, RCA was clearly not as depressive as DNR or doxorubicin.

Experimental Antitumor Activity

Usually, the antitumor activities of RCA were, at *equitoxic doses*, of the same magnitude as those obtained with DNR.

In Ehrlich ascites tumor, the two compounds were inactive on the resistant strain (EAT, R). In a recent study by Bourut and Chenu (I.C.I.G.), a cross-resistance was also observed on a P388/ADM leukemia strain between the following compounds: RCA, carubicin (carminomycin), tetrahydropyranyladriamycin, N-L-leucyl-DNR, 4'-epi-doxorubicin, and aclarubicin (aclacinomycin A). The anthracenedione derivative mitoxantrone was not cross-resistant (unpublished results).

L1210 LEUKEMIA

The therapeutic indexes of RCA and DNR were found to be very close.

AKR-S LEUKEMIA

Against the AKR-S tumor, RCA gave better results than those obtained with DNR (Table 1).

Conclusions

RCA is a semisynthetic anthracycline derivative and the followings were determined by our study:

1. It differs from DNR by the replacement of daunosamine by an aminocyclohexane carboxylic acid linked to the aglycone by an ester bond.
2. Its general toxicity is lower, it has less mutagenic activity, and, above all, it appears to be less cardiotoxic.
3. At equivalent doses, its experimental antitumor activity was close to that of DNR.
4. A cross-resistance was observed between RCA and DNR.

More experimental studies are needed, particularly in pharmacokinetics and pharmacology, before this analogue can be considered for clinical use.

Table 1. AKR-S Leukemia (First Graft of a Spontaneous AKR Leukemia)

Compound	I.P. (mg/kg)	10^6 Cells		10^5 Cells		10^4 Cells	
		T/C × 100	Survivors	T/C × 100	Survivors	T/C × 100	Survivors
RCA	15.0	360	3/10	3/0	2/10	440	7/10
	5.0	146	0/10	200	0/10	426	8/10
	2.5	124	0/10	120	0/10	330	5/10
	1.0	103	0/10	123	0/10	143	1/10
DNR	0.75	117	0/10	110	0/10	300	4/10
	0.25	100	0/10	120	0/10	290	4/10
	0.05	100	0/10	104	0/10	93	0/10

REFERENCES

1. Jollès G, Maral R, Messer M, Ponsinet G: Antitumor activity of daunorubicin derivatives. In *Cancer Chemotherapy II*. Hellman, K, and Connors, TA (eds), Plenum Press, New York, 1976, p. 237.
2. Chabbert V, Vial H: Cytotoxic substances in monolayer tissue cultures by an agar diffusion method. *Exp Cell Res 22, 264, 1961.*
3. Zbinden G, Brandle E: Toxicologic screening of daunorubicin (NSC-82151), adriamycin (NSC-123 127) and their derivatives in rats. *Cancer Chemother Rep 59: 707, 1975.*
4. Dantchev D, Slioussartchouk V, Paintrand M, Hayat M, Bourut C, Mathé, G: Electron microscopic studies of the skin after treatment of golden hamsters with adriamycin, detorubicin, AD 32 and aclacinomycin. *Cancer Treat Rep 63: 1979.*
5. Ames BN, McCann J, Yamasaki E: Methods for detecting carcinogens and mutagens with the Salmonella/mammalian-microsome mutagenicity test. *Mutat Res 31: 347, 1975.*

CHAPTER 32

Antitumor Activity and Cardiac Toxicity of 4'-Deoxydoxorubicin in Mice

A. M. Casazza

After the isolation and characterization of daunorubicin and doxorubicin (DOX) and the detection of the high antitumor activity of these compounds clinically, a program was undertaken at Farmitalia Carlo Erba to detect new anthracyclines having higher antitumor activity and lower toxicity in comparison with the parent drugs. Out of the several derivatives synthesized and investigated,[1] compounds bearing modifications at position 4' of the amino sugar showed particularly interesting properties.[5] The compounds belonging to this group that have been studied more in depth are: 4'-epiDOX, 4'-O-methy1DOX and 4'-deoxyDOX. The first compound, 4'-epiDOX, has already entered clinical trial and is now in phase II evaluation, as has been discussed (Bonedonna and Bonfante) in this book. 4'-O-Methy1DOX showed a very peculiar higher effectiveness than DOX against L1210 leukemia in mice. The last compound of this small series, 4'-deoxy-DOX, presented very striking biologic properties, which are summarized in this report.

Chemical synthesis, biochemical properties, and preliminary data on the cytotoxicity and antitumor activity of 4'-deoxy-DOX have been reported in 1976.[2] Some biochemical and pharmaco-kinetic properties are reported in Table 1. 4'-Deoxy-DOX was as active as DOX on DNA and RNA polymerases, and it equally bound to DNA; a slight but significant difference was observed in the pKa_1 on the molecule; the higher partition coefficient in N-butanol/ 0.01 M-tris sodium chloride buffer, and the higher cell uptake could account for the higher cytotoxicity in comparison with DOX against in vitro cell cultures.[6]

The cytotoxicity data that were first reported were obtained on a HeLa cell subline that was extremely sensitive to some new derivatives; more recent data indicate that 4'-deoxyDOX is about twice as toxic as DOX on HeLa cells. Against ascitic leukemias, 4'-deoxyDOX administered I.P. was as active as DOX[5] and slightly more potent. When administered I.V., 4'-deoxyDOX proved to be more toxic and more potent than DOX. For example, in mice bearing Gross leukemia treated daily for 3 days I.V., the optimal dose of 4'-deoxyDOX was 2.25–2.75 mg/kg (T/C%:233), while the optimal dose of DOX was 5.5 mg/kg (T/C%:216).[5] 4'-DeoxyDOX was fully investigated against a large number of solid tumors, both human tumors transplanted in nude mice[10,11] and mouse tumors transplanted in conventional mice.[4,12] The most interesting results coming from these studies are summarized in Tables 2–4. The compounds were given I.V. every week for a total of 4 weeks, starting when the tumor was palpable. Only the results obtained at the optimal dose are reported here.

Table 2 reports the data obtained against human melanomas transplanted in nude

Farmitalia Carlo Erba Research Laboratories, Nerviano, Milano, Italy

Table 1.   Effects on *in Vitro* Systems[a]

	ID$_{50}$ (μM) Polymerases		Kapp · 10^{-6}			L1210 Uptake	HeLa ID$_{50}$
Compound	RNA	DNA	(M^{-1})	pKa	P	%	(nM)
DOX	6	12	3.3	8.3	6.5	100	310
4'-DeoxyDOX	6	10	3.3	8.6	15.0	240	17

[a]Data from Di Marco et al.[6]

mice, and the mouse melanoma B16, injected S.C. In all these systems, it is peculiar to observe the high effectiveness of DOX, which is known as not being active in melanoma patients, and the fact that 4'-deoxyDOX was less active than DOX.

Table 3 reports the data obtained against human mammary carcinomas transplanted into nude mice and against the spontaneus mammary carcinoma of C3H female mice at the third transplant. These tumors were highly sensitive to DOX activity, in good correlation with the clinical data. 4'-DeoxyDOX showed also a very good antitumor activity, but some tumors were less sensitive to 4'-deoxyDOX than to DOX. Table 4 reports the data obtained against human colon adenocarcinomas transplanted into nude mice and against two colon tumors of conventional mice: the undifferentiated carcinoma 26 and the adenocarcinoma 38. The effectiveness of DOX was definitely lower than that exerted against highly sensitive mammary carcinoma, and only two tumors were inhibited by >50%. Conversely all the colon

tumors tested were inhibited by >50% by the new derivative 4'-deoxyDOX, and the two tumors whose growth was reduced by DOX by >50% (the human tumor T 219 and the mouse tumor 38) were inhibited by 4'-deoxyDOX by 90% or more.

In conclusion, these data show that 4'-deoxyDOX is a peculiar new anthracycline derivative, showing a different spectrum of antitumor activity in comparison with DOX. Besides this very interesting and stimulating property, 4'-deoxyDOX was shown to be very promising also when investigated from the toxicological point of view.

The cardiac toxicity of this compound was the object of several studies carried out in two animal species, the mouse and the rabbit. The data regarding the toxic effects in rabbits treated chronically I.V. have been already reported.

At the highest dose tested (0.525 mg/kg/day), 4'-deoxyDOX was lethal in 100% of the animals, probably because of the high hematologic impairment. At the intermediate dose tested (0.3 mg/kg/day)

Table 2.   Effect Against Melanomas

	% Inhibition of Tumor Growth			
	Human[a]			Mouse[b]
Compound	T 242	T 354	T 355	B16
DOX[c]	87	56	51	95
4'-DeoxyDOX[d]	76	42	33	83

[a]Data from Giuliani et al.[10]
[b]Data from Casazza et al.[4]
[c]Optimal dose: 10 mg/kg I.V., every 7 days for four times.
[d]Optimal dose: 6 mg/kg I.V., every 7 days for four times.

Table 3.   Effect Against Mammary Carcinomas

	% Inhibition			
	Human[a]			Mouse[a]
Compound	T 112	T 378	T 386	C3H
DOX[b]	88	96	90	−72[c]
4'-DeoxyDOX[d]	93	65	67	−52

[a]See Table 2.
[b]Optimal dose (mg/kg): 10 in nude mice, 7.5 in C3H mice.
[c]% regression of tumor volume.
[d]Optimal dose (mg/kg): 6 in nude mice, 6.25 in C3H mice.

Table 4. Effect Against Colon Carcinomas

| | % Inhibition of Tumor Growth | | | | | |
| | Human[a] | | | | Mouse[b] | |
Compound	T 183	T 219	T 374	T 380	26	38
DOX[c]	19	63[d]	44	33	52	67
4'-DeoxyDOX[e]	65	> 99	72	59	67	90

[a]Data from Giuliani et al.[11]
[b]Data from Casazza et al.[4] and Savi et al.[12]
[c]Optimal dose (mg/kg): 10 in nude mice, 6 in conventional mice.
[d]At 6.6 mg/kg.
[e]Optimal dose (mg/kg): 6 in nude mice, 4 in conventional mice.

thrombocytopenia was observed. The most interesting finding of this study was the complete lack of histhologically detectable cardiac lesions in the rabbits treated with 4'-deoxyDOX at tolerated and at toxic doses; conversely, the repeated treatment with DOX provoked serious cardiac lesions and the percentage of animals with lesions was dose dependent.

Studies in mice have been carried out in two different strains: the CD 1 mice[5] and the C3H mice.[3,4] CD 1 mice were treated I.V. 10 times according to the following schedule: 2 treatments/week for 5 weeks, with a 2-week interval between the second and the third week of treatment to allow

recovery of the bone marrow depression. The results of previous and more recent studies are reported in Table 5. Treatment with DOX caused the appearance at distance (the mice were killed 1 month after the last treatment) of cardiac lesions that from the daily dose of 2 mg/kg on, were present in all the animals, and involved both the atrium and the ventricles, the degree of severity was dose dependent. However, the treatment with 4'-deoxy-DOX caused light lesions only in one of five mice treated with 1.3 mg/kg, and in one of five mice treated with 2.6 mg/kg.

An interesting study was carried out in C3H mice. We have here evaluated the cardiac lesions caused by the treatment, both in mice bearing the mammary carcinoma tumor, in which the antitumor activity was evaluated and in normal mice treated in parallel.

This method, recently set up in our laboratories, allows the detection of antitumor activity and cardiac toxicity in the same animals, presenting therefore advantages in respect to previously reported methodologies. The results of this particular study, presented in Table 6, show that at active doses DOX was cardiotoxic, whereas 4'-deoxyDOX at active doses induced only scattered, nondose-dependent lesions.

Table 5. Cardiac Toxicity in CD1 Mice[a]

| | | Left Atrium | | | Ventricles | | | |
Compound	Dose (mg/kg/day)	No.	% with Lesions	Grade	No.	% with Lesions	Grade	% Deaths
DOX	1	10	40	0.2	15	50	0.3	0
		7	0	0	8	25	0.16	20
	2	10	100	0.8	15	100	2.1	0
	4	10	100	6.4	15	100	6.2	10
		4	100	4.5	4	100	1.2	60
4'-DeoxyDOX	0.32	5	0	0	5	0	0	0
	0.65	5	0	0	5	0	0	0
	1.3	5	20	0.1	5	20	0.1	0
		5	0	0	5	0	0	
	2.6	5	20	0.2	5	0	0	10
	5.2		n.d.			n.d.		100

[a]Data from Casazza et al.[4] and from Bellini, O. (unpublished).

Table 6. Evaluation of Antitumor Activity and Cardiac Toxicity in Mice Bearing Mammary Carcinoma, or in Normal Mice Treated in Parallel

Drug	Dose (mg/kg)[a]	Mice with Tumor			Normal Mice		
		Tumor Growth (+) or Regression (−) %	Heart Lesions[b]			Heart Lesions	
			A	V	Toxic Deaths	A	V
		+ 866	0	0.3	0/10	0.1	0.2
DOX	6	− 21	0.9	3.6	0/10	0.7	1.2
	7.5	− 72	1.3	4.0	0/10	1.7	2.0
	9.3	− 82	1.4	4.8	7/10	2.4	3.6
4'-DeoxyDOX	4	+ 97	0.2	0.3	0/10	0	0
	5	− 31	0.3	0.5	0/10	0.1	0.3
	6.25	− 52	0	0.5	0/10	0	0.3

[a]Given I.V. every 7 days for four times.
[b]A: atrium; V: ventricle.

In summary, it can be concluded that 4'-deoxyDOX is a new anthracycline that is not cardiotoxic in mice and rabbits and is selectively more active than DOX against colon carcinomas.

The reasons for these peculiar characteristics are still a matter of speculation. 4'-DeoxyDOX has a higher rate of elimination than DOX from mouse tissues, and particularly from the heart[9] and this may be *one* of the reasons for the lower cardiotoxicity of this new analogue compared with its parent compound (other mechanisms are presently being investigated in several laboratories). Also a parallel can be seen between higher acute toxicity and higher drug levels of 4'-deoxyDOX versus DOX in the spleen. The differences between these two compounds with regard to general toxicity and cardiac toxicity can be partly explained by the differences in pharmacokinetic.[7] This does not seem to be the case for the selectively different antitumor effect observed,[8] since equal drug levels in colon tumors were observed after administration of DOX and 4'-deoxyDOX. Several studies are in progress in our laboratory in order to characterize such activities better, and to find an explanation for these very interesting and stimulating differences.

REFERENCES

1. Arcamone F: The development of new antitumor anthracyclines. In *Anticancer Agents Based on Natural Product Models*. Academic Press, New York 1980, pp 1–41.
2. Arcamone F, Penco S, Redaelli S: Synthesis and antitumor activity of 4'-deoxydoxorubicin and 4'-deoxyadriamycin. *J Med Chem* 19: 1424–1425, 1976.
3. Bellini O, Savi G, Casazza AM: Investigations on the antitumor activity and cardiotoxicity of anthracyclines in C3H mice. *Proceedings of the 12th International Congress of Chemotherapy, Florence, Italy*, July 19–24, 1981.
4. Casazza AM, Bellini O, Savi G, Di Marco A: Antitumor activity and cardiac toxicity of 4'-deoxydoxorubicin (4'-deoxyDX) in mice. *Proc Am Assoc Cancer Res* 22: 267, 1981.
5. Casazza AM, Di Marco A, Bonadonna G, Bonfante V, Bertazzoli C, Bellini O, Pratesi G, Sala L, Ballerini L: Effect of modifications in position 4 of the chromophore or in position 4' of the aminosugar on the antitumor activity and toxicity of daunorubicin and doxorubicin. In *Anthracyclines: Current Status and New Developments*. Crooke ST, Reich SD, (Eds), Academic Press, New York, 1980, pp 403–430.
6. Di Marco A, Casazza AM, Dasdia T, Necco A, Pratesi G, Rivolta P, Velcich A, Zaccara A, Zunino F: Changes of activity of daunorubicin, adriamycin and stereoisomers following the introduction or removal of hydroxyl group in the amino sugar moiety. *Chem Biol Interact* 19: 291-302, 1977.
7. Formelli F, Casazza, AM: Relationships between tissue distribution and toxicity of new anthracyclines in mice. *Proceedings of the 12th International Congress of Chemotherapy, Florence, Italy*, July 19–24, 1981.
8. Formelli F, Fumagalli A, Giuliani F, Casazza AM,

Kaplan NO: Tissue distribution of Doxorubicin (DX) and 4'-deoxydoxorubicin (4'-deoxyDX) in nude and conventional mice bearing colon tumors. *Proc Am Assoc Cancer Res 22: 267, 1981.*

9. Formelli F, Pollini C, Casazza AM, Di Marco A, Mariani A: Fluorescence assays and pharmacokinetic studies of 4'-deoxydoxorubicin and doxorubicin in organs of mice bearing solid tumors. *Cancer Chemother Pharmacol 5: 139–144, 1981.*

10. Giuliani FC, Coirin AK, Rice MR, Kaplan NO: Effect of 4'-doxorubicin analogs on heterotransplantation of human tumors in congenitally athymic mice. *Cancer Treat Rep. 65:1063–1075, 1981.*

11. Giuliani FC, Kaplan NO: New doxorubicin analogs active against doxorubicin resistant colon tumor xenografts in the nude mouse. *Cancer Res 40: 4682–4687, 1980.*

12. Savi G, Casazza AM, Giuliani, F: Attività di 4'-desossidoxorubicina su tumori del colon murini, e studi di terapia combinata con 5 fluorouracile. *Tumori 67 (Suppl 2): 183, 1981.*

CHAPTER 33

QRS-T Effects of Doxorubicin and N,N-Dibenzyl Daunorubicin in the Rat

R. A. Jensen, E. M. Acton, and J. H. Peters

Cancer chemotherapy with the anthracyclines doxorubicin (DOX) and daunorubicin (DNR) is limited by a dose-dependent cardiomyopathy and risk of the irreversible development of congestive heart failure as treatment progresses.[2,6] As a result, new anthracyclines that combine good antitumor activity with low cardiotoxicity are widely sought. However, development of anthracycline analogues is severely hampered by the lack of a validated test method specifically for chronic cardiotoxicity, despite the intense concern with this problem for nearly 10 years and numerous studies using various approaches, both with isolated tissue and with animals.

Zbinden and co-workers[14,15] have used the rat electrocardiogram (ECG) as a model system for evaluating the cardiotoxicity of anthracyclines. They have shown that administration of DOX and other anthracyclines in multiple doses causes a progressive widening of the QRS complex. More recently, Buyniski and Hirth[5] described a rat ECG test system that was based on anthracycline-induced reductions in QRS voltage. However, the relation between ECG changes and myocardial damage in the rat has not been conclusively established.

We have recently restudied the effects of DOX on the rat ECG, focusing on DOX-induced changes in the duration of both the QRS complex and the QαT interval.[10] In addition, we investigated transmembrane potential changes as well as changes in isometric contractile activity and histopathologic alterations in cardiac tissue preparations taken from the same DOX-treated rats in an attempt to correlate ECG changes with electrical, mechanical, and structural abnormalities on the cellular level. The results of the DOX study have been incorporated in a new ECG model for cardiotoxicity that is essentially an extension of the Zbinden test. It is based upon the assumption that persistent QRS-T interval changes (i.e., alterations in ventricular activation and recovery time) reflect structural damage or membrane changes leading to structural damage in the myocardium.

This report presents a description of the comparative cardiotoxicity of DOX and the analogue N,N-dibenzyldaunorubicin (B$_2$D, synthesized at SRI) using this model system. B$_2$D was chosen for study because it was 31% more efficacious than DOX against P388 mouse leukemia (dosed every 4, 5, 9, 13 days; tumor cells/controls [T/C] = 209% versus 160%). Compared to DOX, B$_2$D required higher doses for antitumor activity (e.g., 5- to 30-fold against mouse P388, depending on schedule). We conclude that B$_2$D warrants further evaluation as a potentially less cardiotoxic agent.

Life Sciences Division SRI International, Menlo Park, California

Materials and Methods

EXPERIMENTAL GROUPS

Female Sprague-Dawley rats with a starting weight of 180-210 g were used in this study. To document overall good health, the animals were observed for 10 days prior to drug administration. During this time, baseline ECGs were recorded and the rats were familiarized with a restraining device.

DOX was obtained from the National Cancer Institute and B_2D was synthesized at SRI.[14] Both drugs were suspended in a 2:1 mixture of polyethylene glycol-200 and isotonic saline. The drug solutions were made fresh daily.

DOX was administered intraperitoneally (I.P.) to three treatment groups (10 rats per group) as follows: Group A, 4 mg/kg daily for 5 days; Group B, 1 mg/kg five times per week for 4 weeks; Group C, 2 mg/kg five times per week for 2 weeks. Therefore the total cumulative dose for each treatment group was 20 mg/kg. Three control groups (5-10 per group) received I.P. injections of the vehicle. The Group B rats were observed for 8-14 weeks after the end of treatment and sacrificed for isolated tissue study[10] at the time signs of congestive heart failure were well developed. All other DOX rats were sacrificed at the end of the treatment schedule.

B_2D was also given to three treatment groups (10 rats per group) : Group D, 10 mg/kg intravenously (I.V.) five times per week for 4 weeks; Group E, 10 mg/kg I.P. five times per week for 6 weeks; Group F, 20 mg/kg I.V. five times per week for 3 weeks. The Group D and Group F rats were observed for 6 to 8 months after the end of treatment for signs of cardiotoxicity.

ECG RECORDINGS AND ANALYSIS

Three to six baseline ECGs were recorded prior to drug administration. During the treatment period, ECG recordings were obtained daily just prior to dosing

(20-24 hours after the previous dose of DOX or B_2D). ECGs were recorded from Group B, Group D, and Group F rats one to two times per week through the post-treatment period. For ECG recordings, the unanesthetized rats were restrained in the ventral position in a small plastic holder, and subcutaneous pin electrodes were positioned over the right scapula and lumbar vertebrae. This bipolar configuration (lead $D^{5,15}$) provides ECG patterns similar to those recorded with the electrodes on the limb extremities (lead II). The amplified signal (Grass P511) was displayed on a Tektronix 502A oscilloscope and photographed with a C-12 oscilloscope camera. For accurate measurements of the electrocardiographic intervals (QRS and QαT), the signal was fed into a LINC-8 computer (or, more recently, a DEC MINC-11). Using a program developed in our laboratory, signal averaging was carried out on 100 ECG signals fitting a noise rejection profile. The composite waveform was stored on tape and subsequently retrieved for analysis via printout on a Hewlett-Packard X-Y plotter. The horizontal sweep of the plotter was set at 0.5 msec/mm. Figure 1 shows photographs of oscilloscope sweeps and Figure 2 provides a comparison of the oscilloscope display and computer-averaged signals. The actual measurements of the ECG intervals were performed on the average signal sequence as follows (see the top trace in Figure 3): 1) the isoelectric line was established as the stable baseline preceding the ascending limb of the R-wave (in the rat ECG, a prominent Q-wave is usually lacking); 2) the duration of the QRS complex was taken as the interval (in milliseconds) from the onset of the pronounced concavity at the start of the R wave to the intersection of the isoelectric line and the ascending limb of the S wave; 3) the duration of the QαT segment was measured as the interval (in milliseconds) between the start of the R wave and the apex of the T wave, in accordance with Lepeschkin[11]

A. RAT 19-1

| PRE-TREATMENT | 8 mg/kg DXR + 24 Hrs | 16 mg/kg DXR + 24 Hrs | 20 mg/kg DXR + 48 Hrs |

B. RAT 20-5

┌──── PRE-TREATMENT ────┐   ┌─ 20 mg/kg DXR + 48 Hrs ─┐

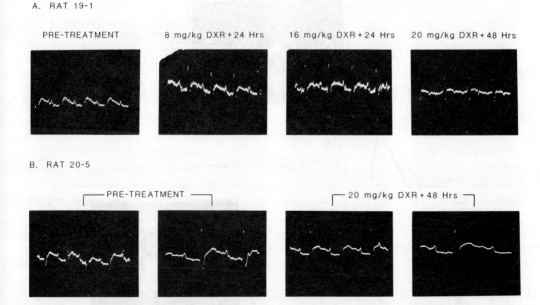

FIGURE 1. Photographs of oscilloscope sweeps showing ECG effects (lead D) of a high-dose DOX on two rats treated with 4 mg/kg I.P. for 5 consecutive days. Oscilloscope sweep speed was 50 msec/cm except in second and fourth photographs in bottom row, where it was 25 msec/cm. Vertical calibration is 250 μV/cm. Terminal ECGs (20 mg/kg plus 24 hours) for both rats were taken immediately before sacrifice for isolated tissue study.

and Buschmann et al.[4] In the rat ECG, the $Q\alpha T$ interval differs from the Q-T interval in that it does not include the flat descending limb of the T wave. This slowly descending T wave, which usually merges into the P wave, makes it difficult to identify the end of the Q-T interval with any accuracy.[1,3,9] Based on the findings of Beinfield and Lehr[1] and Buschmann et al.[4] no attempts were made to correct the $Q\alpha T$ interval for changes in heart rate in this study. Drug-induced changes in QRS and $Q\alpha T$ durations were determined for individual rats in terms of prolongation (in milliseconds) over the pretreatment value (mean of two or three determinations). The mean changes were then established for the treatment group and plotted as a function of dose and time. Comparisons were done between the pretreatment QRS and $Q\alpha T$ values and subsequent DOX responses by means of the t test for paired data.

Results

ECG CHANGES ASSOCIATED WITH DOX TREATMENT

The effects of treatment with a high dose of DOX (Group A rats, 4 mg/kg × 5 I.P.) on the rat ECG, as measured conventionally via oscilloscope display and with the computer-averaging technique, are illustrated in Figures 1 to 3. With increasing cumulative dose, the earliest (and most consistent) change observed was a prolongation in the $Q\alpha T$ interval (defined in the top trace of Figure 3). $Q\alpha T$ prolongation was comprised primarily of a lengthening of the $S\alpha T$ segment and in 8 of 10 rats was accompanied by a progressive flattening of the T wave. The $Q\alpha T$ changes were soon followed by a progressive and asymmetric widening of the QRS complex (wherein prolongation in the duration of the S wave exceeded that of the R wave) and a marked increase, followed by a de-

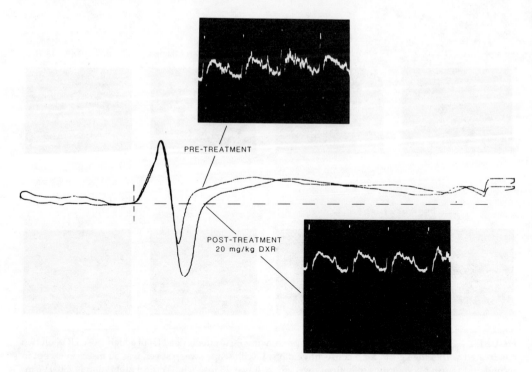

FIGURE 2. Comparison of computer-averaged ECG tracings with conventional oscilloscope displays. Group A rat (4 mg/kg × 5 I.P.). Computer tracings represent 100 cardiac cycles. Photographs display ECG signals before computer averaging. The superimposed tracings reveal that 24 hours after the end of DOX treatment, the following QRS-T changes had occurred: 1) the QRS complex was prolonged by an increase in the duration of the S wave, with no change in the duration of the R wave; 2) the QαT interval had been prolonged primarily by an increase in the duration of the SαT segment; 3) the amplitude of the R wave was unchanged, whereas that of the S wave was markedly increased; and 4) there was only a slight decrease in the amplitude of the T wave. These changes are somewhat atypical in that DOX treatment usually produces a slight prolongation in the duration of the R wave as well as T wave flattening. No attempts were made in this study to quantify changes in QRS-T voltages or changes in R, S, and SαT durations. The QRS and QαT durations are defined in the top trace in Figure 3.

crease, in the deflection of the S wave. Changes in the amplitude of the R wave were inconsistent — in some rats it showed an increase followed by a decrease, but in others it was unchanged. Results similar to these were obtained with the Group B (1 mg/kg × 20 I.P.) and Group C (2 mg/kg × 10 I.P.) rats, and the magnitude of change in a given parameter (with the exception of the R wave) appeared to be related to cumulative dose.

Figure 4 graphically illustrates the mean changes in QRS and QαT durations with respect to pretreatment values as a function of dose and time for the Group A and Group B rats. At the end of treatment in both groups of rats (signified by the vertical dashed line), the QRS and QαT durations are markedly increased compared with pretreatment values and with those recorded from control animals. Figure 4B demonstrates that during a 4- to 18-week posttreatment period in the low-dose group, the prolongation in the QRS complex tends to reverse, but that of the QαT interval does not. The QRS reversal is characterized by a progressive loss of the S wave until very little S wave deflection remains, as well as the appearance of a spike-shaped R wave. Thus, describing

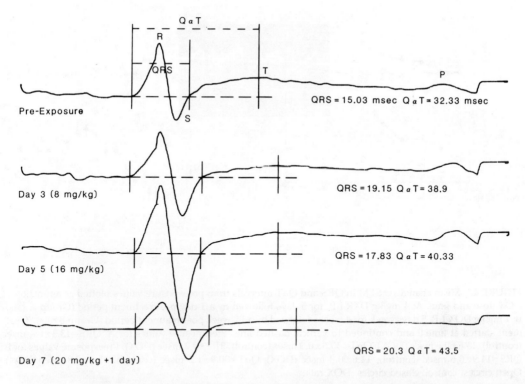

FIGURE 3.   Effect of DOX treatment (4 mg/kg × 5 I.P.) on the duration of the QRS complex and QαT interval. ECG components identified in top trace. Each trace represents a computer-generated average of 100 cardiac cycles. Treatment ECGs (days 3, 5, and 7) recorded 24 hours after dosing (cumulative dose indicated). DOX treatment in this rat caused a prolongation in the QRS complex and QαT interval, an increase followed by a decrease in the R wave and S wave deflections, and a flattening of the T wave. With progressive T wave flattening, accurate measurement of the QαT interval becomes more difficult.

this phenomenon as a QRS reversal may be misleading because the original waveform does not reappear. The mean QRS and QαT changes observed in the Group B rats both during and following DOX treatment are also shown in Table 1.

When viewed in the context of the *in vitro* transmembrane potential findings[10] the irreversibility of the QαT changes and the uniqueness of the changes in the QRS complex suggest that both may be utilized as markers of ECG cardiotoxicity in the rat model. To quantify the effects of different anthracycline compounds on the rat ECG, we have established an index of cardiotoxicity termed the Δ-10 dose. This is the cumulative dose at which the following criteria are satisfied: 1) mean QRS and

QαT prolongation of at least 10% of the pretreatment level is achieved, 2) the prolongation observed is significant with respect to pretreatment mean values at the $p < 0.05$ level, and 3) both of the foregoing are maintained through two successive observations. The Δ-10 doses recorded for DOX in the three groups of rats evaluated in this study are provided in Table 2. The Δ-10 dose for QRS widening was 8 mg/kg in Groups A and C and 9 mg/kg in Group B. The Δ-10 dose for QαT prolongation was 4 mg/kg in all three groups.

ECG CHANGES ASSOCIATED WITH B_2D TREATMENT

B_2D was administered I.V. in two experiments (Groups D and F) and I.P. in one ex-

A
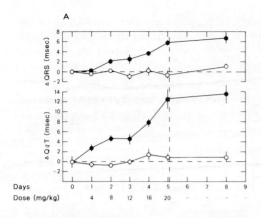

B
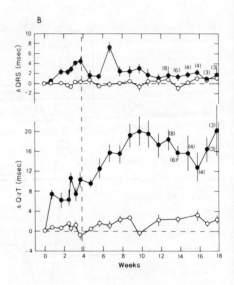

FIGURE 4. Mean changes ±SEM in QRS and QαT intervals from preexposure values plotted as a function of DOX dose and time. A: 4 mg/kg DXR I.P. for 5 days followed by a 3-day posttreatment period (Group A rats). B: 1 mg/kg DOX I.P. 5 days/week for 4 weeks followed by a 14-week posttreatment period (Group B rats). Treatment started at time 0 and continued to vertical dashed line. Preexposure values for A: QRS=13.3±0.4 msec (control), 13.6±0.6 msec (DOX); QαT=30.6±0.9 msec (control), 31.2±0.2 msec (DOX). Preexposure values for B: QRS=14.9±0.6 msec (control), 14.6±0.3 msec (DOX); QαT=30.9±1.2 msec (control), 31.0±0.8 msec (DOX). Open circles: control; closed circles: DOX rats.

periment (Group E). ECG changes occurred when the drug was given by both routes. Based on distribution studies, however, we consider the I.V. route to be the most reliable (Peters *et al.*, unpublished observations).

Although the dose requirements differed greatly, the QRS-T effects of B₂D were similar to those exerted by DOX. Fig-

ure 5 provides a direct comparison of the results obtained with the Group B rats (DOX, 1 mg/kg × 20 I.P.) and Group D rats (B₂D 10 mg/kg × 20 I.V.). At the termination of dosing in the Group D experiment (200 mg/kg cumulative dose), there was only a modest prolongation in the QαT interval and flattening of the T wave, both of which reversed during the post-

Table 1. QRS and QαT Effects of DOX (1 mg/kg × 20, I.P.) for Group B Rats[a]

Dose (mg/ kg)	Pre-treat-ment	Change from Pretreatment					(mean ± SEM)				
		4	9	11	15	19	20 +1 week	20 +4 weeks	20 +6 weeks	20 +12 weeks	20 +14 weeks
ΔQRS (msec)	14.98 ±0.41	0.74 ±0.79	2.52 ±0.62	2.4 ±5.1	2.91 ±0.49	4.08 ±0.59	4.58 ±0.86	2.07 ±0.96	3.05 ±0.35	2.15 ±1.2	1.80
p	—	NS	0.02	0.005	0.005	0.001	0.001	0.05	0.02	0.01	NS
ΔQαT (msec)	30.9 ±0.86	3.10 ±1.61	6.43 ±1.0	6.19 ±1.15	7.14 ±1.25	10.22 ±0.73	9.77 ±1.69	15.69 ±2.81	21.29 ±2.99	12.78 ±5.2	20.8
p	—	0.005	0.005	0.001	0.001	0.001	0.001	0.001	0.001	0.025	0.02

[a]Six of 8 rats developed signs of congestive heart failure (and *in vitro* signs of contractile failure and structural damage).

Table 2. Cumulative Doses in mg/kg Where Sustained

Group	QRS	QαT
A (DOX 4 × 5 I.P.)	8	4
B (DOX 1 × 20 I.P.)	9	4
C (DOX 2 × 10 I.P.)	8	4
D (B₂D 10 × 20 I.V.)	N/A[a]	180
E (B₂D 10 × 30 I.P.)	240	170
F (B₂D 20 × 15 I.V.)	280	180

[a]10% Widening never occurred for these rats.

treatment period. The changes observed at 20 mg/kg cumulative dose DOX by contrast, were irreversible. Figure 6 shows the results obtained with the Group F rats (20 mg/kg × 15 I.V.). At 280 mg/kg cumulative dose, the QαT and T wave changes were more pronounced and a prolongation in the QRS complex had occurred. Even after 300 mg/kg had been administered, however, the QRS and QαT changes reversed during the posttreatment period. At the end of an 8-month posttreatment observation, the ECGs recorded from the Group D rats were normal.

The mean QRS and QαT effects of B₂D observed in the Group F rats are presented in Table 3, and the Δ-10 doses calculated in all three B₂D experiments are listed in Table 2. The Δ-10 dose for QαT lengthening is very consistent from experiment to experiment. These results show that the total doses of B₂D (200 and 300 mg/kg)

were approximately 50–75 times the dose of DOX for significant threshold effects on QαT that denote cardiotoxicity. The total B₂D doses are also 25–38 times the dose of DOX for significant threshold effects of QRS that denote cardiotoxicity. The B₂D Δ-10 doses are 30–35 and 42–45 times the DOX Δ-10 doses for QRS and QαT prolongation, respectively.

POSTTREATMENT MORBIDITY AND MORTALITY

Six of eight Group B rats (DOX 1mg/kg × 20 I.P.) developed signs of congestive heart failure during the posttreatment period (8–14 weeks after the end of dosing). At the time heart failure occurred, the QαT interval was markedly prolonged and the T wave substantially decreased. Hearts taken from these animals revealed contraction abnormalities as well as significant structural damage.[10] By contrast, the Group D and Group F rats (200 and 300 mg/kg B₂D) survived with no signs of heart failure and with normal ECGs until they were sacrificed 6–8 months after the end of treatment.

Discussion

We have demonstrated that both DOX and B₂D cause a dose-dependent prolongation in the QRS complex and the QαT interval in the rat ECG, and using the Δ-10 doses as indices of comparative activity, we conclude that B₂D is at least 30–45

Table 3. QRS and QαT Effects of B₂D (20 mg/kg × 15, I.V.) for Group F Rats[a]

Dose (mg/kg)	Pre-treatment	80	100	180	200	240	280	300 + 3 weeks	300 + 8 weeks
					Change from Pretreatment				
ΔQRS (msec)	15.1	0.07 ±0.23	−0.02 ±0.22	0.26 ±0.38	−0.26 ±0.40	0.94 ±0.45	1.94 ±0.61	−0.34 ±0.53	0.13 ±0.59
p	—	NS	NS	NS	NS	NS	0.02	NS	NS
ΔQαT (msec)	32.1	1.59 ±0.81	1.93 ±0.49	3.99 ±0.56	3.27 ±0.74	4.68 ±1.89	5.67 ±1.54	1.11 ±1.02	1.17 ±0.61
p	—	NS	0.005	0.001	0.005	0.05	0.01	NS	NS

[a]All rats survived with no signs of heart failure and with normal ECGs at the time of sacrifice.

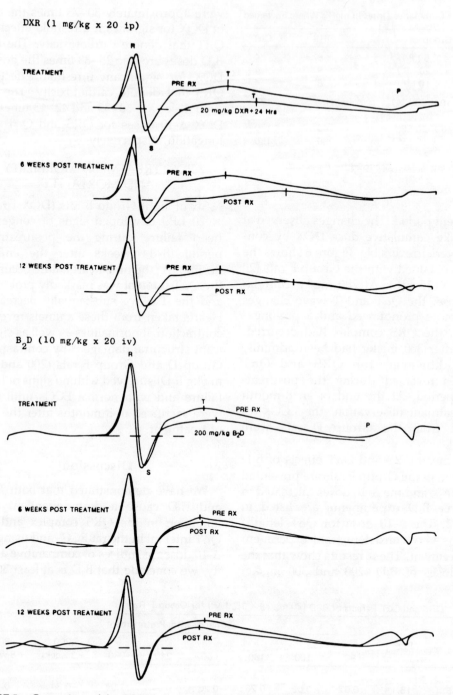

FIGURE 5. Comparison of the QRS-T effects of DOX (top, Group B rat, 1 mg/kg×20 I.P.) with those of B₂D (bottom, Group D rat, 10×20 mg/kg I.V.). Each tracing represents a computer-generated average of 100 cardiac cycles. Each pair represents a posttreatment record (24 hours, 6 weeks, and 12 weeks) superimposed on a pretreatment tracing. The DOX treated rat developed congestive heart failure shortly before the 12-week record was obtained. In this animal DOX caused a marked prolongation in the QRS and QαT intervals which did not reverse following the end of treatment. The B₂D treated rat survived with a normal ECG.

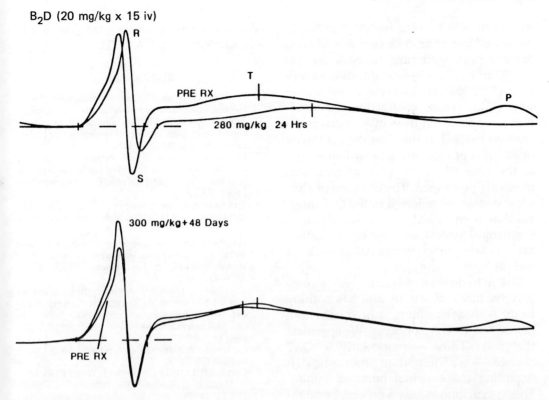

FIGURE 6. QRS-T effects of B_2D (Group F rat, 20 mg/kg × 15 I.V.). Treatment and posttreatment records superimposed on pretreatment tracings. Increasing the cumulative dose of B_2D from 200 to 300 mg/kg (see Fig. 5) caused QRS and QαT prolongation which reversed to normal 48 days after the end of treatment. All Group F rats survived with normal ECGs at the time of sacrifice 8 months after the end of treatment.

times less active than DOX in causing QRS-T changes suggestive of cardiotoxicity.

The duration of the QRS complex in the ECG represents the time required for activation of the ventricular myocardium, and the QαT interval is reflective of the duration of electrical systole and the rate of ventricular repolarization. Clearly the rates of activation and recovery are prolonged in DOX- and B_2D-treated rats. At the doses studied, however, the changes induced by B_2D are reversible, whereas those caused by DOX are not. The ECG changes observed for DOX as well as B_2D persist well after elimination of the drug from the body: therefore they must be attributed to structural modifications in the myocardium.

The model system described in this re-

port was developed by comparing the QRS-T effects of DOX with transmembrane potential, contractile, and structural changes in ventricular muscle preparations isolated from treated animals.[10] In tissues obtained 24–48 hours after the end of dosing (20 mg/kg cumulative dose) the maximum rate of depolarization ($\dot{V}_{max}$) was substantially reduced (a mean decrease of 30 V/sec) with no change in resting potential, which very likely accounts for QRS prolongation. We also found that action (AP) duration was consistently prolonged by up to 40%, which provides an explanation for the increased duration of the QαT interval. Mechanical studies on preparations obtained 8–14 weeks after termination of dosing revealed the following changes in isometric contractile activity, all of which were highly significant: decreased maximum rate of rise in tension (dT/dt), prolonged time to peak tension (TPT), an increase in total duration of tension (Td), and an increase in relaxation time (TR$_{1/2}$). These contraction abnormalities were recorded from myocardial preparations excised at the time the rat developed signs of congestive heart failure and at the time when the QαT interval was markedly prolonged. The duration of electrical systole, as reflected in the Q-T interval, has been linked to a prolongation in mechanical systole in a variety of pathological states in experimental animals as well as human beings.[13]

The Δ-10 dose is, of course, only a comparative index of activity and has nothing to do with determining if myopathy and failure will or will not occur. We speculate that reversibility — particularly in QαT changes — is an important prognostic sign regarding the eventual onset of failure. This speculation is based on serial evaluations made with DOX and B$_2$D, as reported here, as well as preliminary ECG data obtained with the anthracycline analogues 3'-deamino-3'-(4-morpholinyl) daunorubicin (MRD) 3'-deamino-3'-(4-methoxy-l-piperdinyl) daunorubicin (MEO), N-benzyldaunorubicin (B$_1$D), and N,N-dibenzyl-13-dihydrodoxorubicin (B$_2$A-OL). Irreversible AαT prolongation always occurred in the animals that did not survive dosing.

The applicability of anthracycline-induced QRS-T changes in the rat to clinical treatment has yet to be established. Q-T prolongation and T wave flattening with anthracycline treatment has been mentioned by various authors,[7,8,12] and it is possible — because of recording techniques, or simply because they have been overlooked — that QRS-T interval changes are more prevalent than reported.

ACKNOWLEDGMENTS

The technical assistance of Susan Winslow is greatly appreciated. This study was supported by CA 25711.

REFERENCES

1. Beinfield WH, Lehr D: QRS-T variations in the rat electrocardiogram. Am J Physiol 214: 197, 1968.
2. Blum RM, Carter SK: Adriamycin. A new anticancer drug with significant clinical activity. Ann Intern Med 80: 249–259, 1974.
3. Bonaccorsi A, Franco R, Garattini S, Morselli P, Pita E: Plasma nortriptyline and cardiac responses in young and old rats. Brit J Pharmacol 60: 21–27, 1977.
4. Buschmann G, Schumacher R, Budden R, Kuhl U: Evaluation of the effect of dopamine and other catecholamines on the electrocardiogram and blood pressure of rats by means of on-line biosignal processing. J Cardiovasc Pharmacol 2: 777–795, 1980.
5. Buyniski JP, Hirth RS: Anthracycline cardiotoxicity in the rat. In Anthracyclines: Current Status and New Developments. Crooke ST, Reich SD (Eds), Academic Press, New York, pp 157–170, 1980
6. Carter SK: Adriamycin — A review. J Nat Cancer Inst 55: 1265, 1975.
7. Cortes EP, Lutman G, Wanka J, Wang JJ, Pickren J, Wallace J, Holland JF: Adriamycin (NSC-123127) cardiotoxicity: A clinicopathological correlation. Cancer Chemotherap Rep 6: 215–225, 1975.
8. Gilladoga AC, Manuel C, Tan C, Wollner N, Murphy ML: Cardiotoxicity of Adriamycin (NSC-123127) in children. Cancer Chemotherap Rep 6: 209–214, 1975.
9. Heering H: The electrocardiogram of the conscious and anesthetized rat. Arch Int Pharmacodyn Ther 185: 308–328, 1970.
10. Jensen RA, Acton EA, Peters JH,: QRS-T effects of doxorubicin in the rat: Correlation with in vitro electrical and mechanical effects. In preparation.
11. Lepeschkin E: The configuration of the T wave and the ventricular action potential in different species of animals. Ann NY Acad Sci 127: 170–178, 1965.
12. Nakayama R, Toyoshima H, Tominaga K, Shinkai T: Electrocardiogram of cardiomyopathy induced by Adriamycin. Int Cong Ser Exerpta Medica 470 (Cardiology): 633–638, 1979.
13. Nierenberg DW, Ransil BJ: QαT interval as a clinical indicator of hypercalcemia. Am J Cardiol 44: 243–248, 1979.
14. Tong GL, Wu HY, Smith TH, Henry DW: Synthesis of N-Alkylated Anthracyclines with enhanced efficacy and reduced cardiotoxicity. J Med Chem 22: 912–918, 1979.
15. Zbinden G, Bachmann E, Holderegger C: Model systems for the cardiotoxic effects of anthracyclines. Antibiot Chemother 23: 255–270, 1978.
16. Zbinden G, Brandle E: Toxicologic screening of daunorubicin (NSC-82151), Adriamycin (NSC-123127), and their derivatives in rats. Cancer Chemotherap Rep 59: 707–715, 1975.

Index